STRENGTH
TRAINING
FOR BASEBALL

STRENGTH TRAINING
FOR BASEBALL

Jose Canseco
and
Dave McKay

A Perigee Book

Perigee Books
are published by
The Putnam Publishing Group
200 Madison Avenue
New York, NY 10016
Copyright © 1990 by MBKA, Inc.

Library of Congress Cataloging-in-Publication Data

Canseco, Jose, date.
Strength training for baseball / Jose Canseco and Dave McKay.
p.   cm.
"A Perigee book."
ISBN 0-399-51596-8
1. Baseball—Training. 2. Physical education and training.
3. Stretching exercises. 4. Weight training.   I. McKay, Dave.
II. Title.
GV875.6.C34   1990   89-28340 CIP
613.7'1—dc20

Responsibility for any adverse effects or unforeseen
consequences resulting from the use of any information
contained herein is expressly disclaimed.

Printed in the United States of America
1 2 3 4 5 6 7 8 9 10

This book has been printed on acid-free paper.

CONTENTS

Author Biographies... 7

Foreword by Bill Shannon.................................... 11

General Preparation 13

Stretching 17

Weight Training 55

Use of the Program.. 143

Conclusion... 158

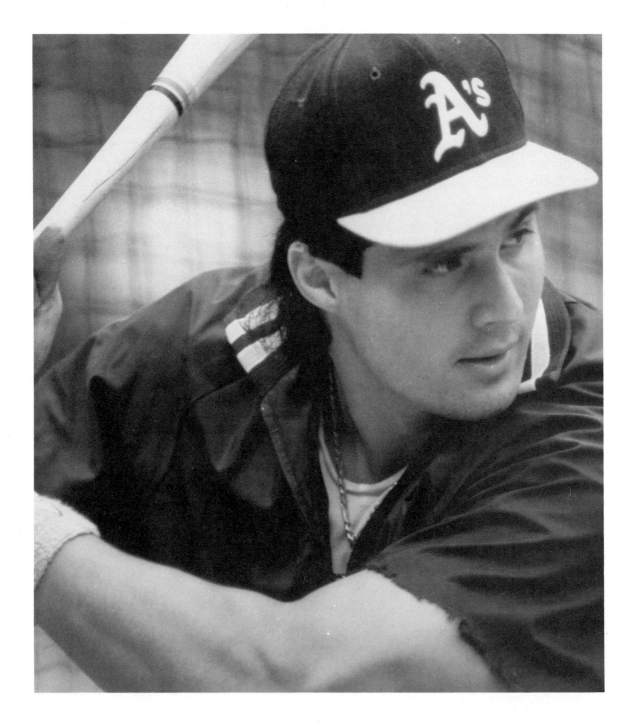

After only three full seasons in the American League, Jose Canseco has established himself as one of the true superstars in the major leagues. In 1988, he became the first player in baseball history to both hit 40 home runs and steal 40 bases in the same season.

When measured against the performance of the greats of the game's long history (Babe Ruth, Rogers Hornsby, Ty Cobb, Lou Gehrig, Henry Aaron, Willie Mays, Mickey Mantle, Stan Musial, Ted Williams, et al.), this is a truly astonishing feat.

Jose Canseco broke into the majors with a smash. He was named Rookie of the Year during his first full season in 1986, when he hit 33 home runs and drove in 117 runs. During the 1988 season, Canseco exceeded both of those figures with 42 home runs and 124 RBI en route to becoming the unanimous choice as the American League Most Valuable Player.

Born in Havana, Cuba, in 1964, Jose Canseco was a fifteenth-round draft choice by the Oakland Athletics in 1982 and, after a slow start in the minor leagues, has become one of the premier players in the illustrious history of the Athletics.

His all-around performance in 1988 (when he batted .307), helped to lift Oakland to the postseason playoffs for the first time in seven years and sent the A's into the World Series for the first time since 1974.

Canseco's dedication and diligence in physical conditioning are legendary even among his peers in major-league baseball.

Dave McKay

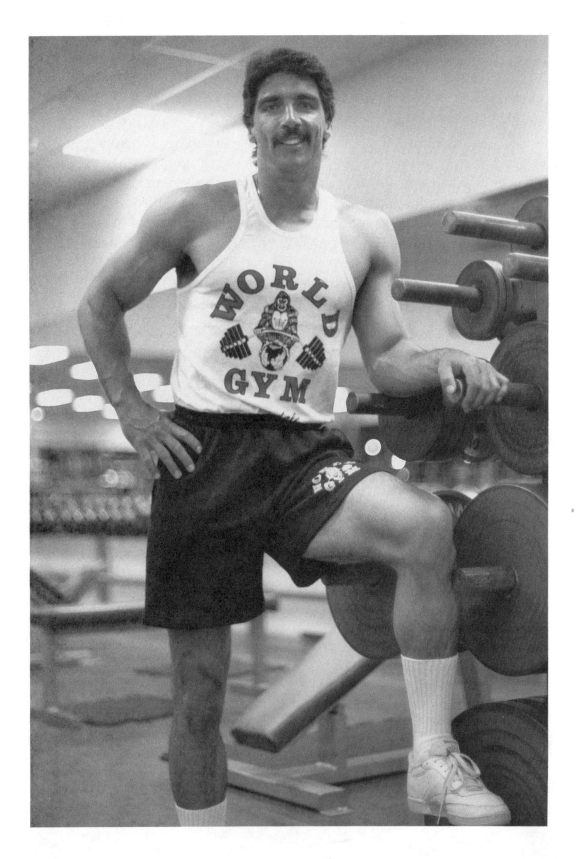

Dave McKay has been a member of the Oakland Athletics organization for more than ten years and is most familiar to A's fans in the Bay Area as the club's first-base coach.

He has a much less visible job as the team's fitness instructor. He is credited with developing the program that has made Oakland the envy of major-league baseball for its physical-conditioning program.

McKay came to the major leagues in 1975 with the Minnesota Twins and hit a home run in his first at bat. He then hit safely in 20 of the next 21 games he played. In 1977, McKay joined the Toronto Blue Jays and was the starting third baseman in the first game ever played by Toronto. In 1978, he tied a major-league record by hitting two doubles in the same inning.

In 1980, McKay joined the Oakland organization as an infielder and has remained with the club since, becoming a coach in 1984.

Born in Vancouver, British Columbia, McKay earned a degree in physical education from Columbia Basin Junior College in Pasco, Washington, then Creighton University, Omaha, Nebraska, before beginning his professional baseball career in 1971.

Acknowledgments

Acknowledgment is due to Tom DiPace for all the photographs
in this book and to Gold's Gym in Scottsdale,
Arizona for providing the photo location.
Thanks are also due to Bill Shannon for his editorial work.

Over the last ten years or so, literally hundreds of workout plans have been marketed in this country, including many specifically designed for sports and potential athletes.

However, few if any of these have struck what seemed to me to be the proper tone for baseball players. Baseball is a sport that requires a wide range of skills, both physical and mental. It is, in brief, a skill game, not a power game.

Despite what one may read or hear about power hitters and power pitchers, it is not sheer size or physical strength that make a successful baseball player. Many fine athletes from other sports have not been notable baseball players.

Part of this, of course, is due to the mental discipline required to play baseball. I have spoken over the years with several top athletes in other sports who have had opportunities to play baseball, and they have all remarked about the mental fatigue of having to go out and play virtually every single day during a 176-day season.

Under the current Basic Agreement, major-league players are entitled to one day off after every 19 played. But in the heat of a pennant race, even this slight respite can go by the board if a prior rainout has to be made up.

Physical conditioning obviously has a major role to play here. By this I mean not just the ability to play through the minor injuries that crop up during the course of a long season, but also stamina and certain types of physical strength. The problem with most conditioning and strength-building programs is that they are not applicable to the needs of baseball players.

This book contains a program designed by a former major leaguer and used successfully by major leaguers. In this regard, it is unique.

Dave McKay was a major-league infielder with the Toronto Blue Jays, the Minnesota Twins, and the Oakland Athletics and now is a coach with the A's. What he has done is create a stretching and workout program that has proven itself in the major leagues. There has been a strong trend in recent years to add a strength coach to the staff of ballclubs. McKay not only coaches first base and performs other on-the-field duties for Oakland, but he is also the team strength coach.

FOREWORD

I don't believe anyone can suggest that the strength program hasn't been effective. It has been used by many of the Oakland players — regulars, reserves, and pitchers alike. Some of the players have been in the majors for many seasons and got into a strength program for the first time when they came to Oakland.

This is clearly the strongest testimony to the value of the program contained in this book — it is used by the men for whom it has been designed and they believe that it has helped them maintain and accelerate their careers.

High on the list of the believers in this program is Jose Canseco. There is no reason here to detail the achievements of Canseco in his major-league career. Suffice it to say that he believes this program has been of material value in assisting him to produce the high level of performance that has made him one of the outstanding players in the majors in a very brief span.

Although Canseco missed the first half of the 1989 season, his performance has been of an all-star caliber — 65 games, 61 hits, 17 home runs and 57 RBIs.

In this book, Jose demonstrates, using more than 150 pictures, the exercises that have helped him improve his body for baseball.

McKay himself shows the reader the proper stretching program in the first half of the book. Both of these programs are identical to those used by the Oakland Athletics, now the dominant team in the American League West.

There is reason to believe that the overall physical condition of the A's has been improved by this program. Perhaps more importantly, it can be used by an aspiring baseball player without fear of harming his chances of attaining the major leagues.

Traditionally, baseball players have shied away from the weight room for fear that overdevelopment may hinder their careers. In this regard, they are generally correct. However, this book addresses that concern directly and delivers a program that a baseball player can follow without fear.

Naturally, exercise and body development alone will not make a major-league player. As mentioned earlier, a lot of elements go into the package that eventually lands a young man in major-league baseball, including discipline and mental toughness as well as skill and a competitive desire.

But this program can certainly give anyone with the other essentials an extra edge.

This book embodies the results of several years of work, investigation, and consultation.

I have discussed and examined the needs of major-league baseball players (as distinct from other athletes and general bodybuilders) with some of the outstanding proponents of bodybuilding in North America. I will mention a couple of them shortly. But first, let's examine the general concept of this book.

Jose Canseco is an outstanding major-league player. Some of the factors that have helped him achieve that status have also helped him in maximizing the value of this program. Jose will never "cheat" on a lift. If he does a lift, he will do it with perfect form technique. I cannot emphasize too much the value of that approach. Perfect form and technique are the only way to go. That is true not only of this program, but any program. If you cheat on a lift, you are only fooling yourself. You will not get the value from the lift that the lift has to give. Other than burning a few calories, you will have gained very little from it. And most important, you will have risked injury.

Jose's demonstrations later in this book are demonstrations of those perfect forms and techniques. It is the way he does his lifts. It is also the *only* way to do the lifts that he demonstrates.

Jose also has a very positive approach to his work. I always tell players to think positively. Tell yourself when you are ready to do your last repetition that it is going to be your best lift, and chances are that it will be. Jose approaches his work exactly that way, which is just one of the things that have made him a model achiever in the program.

When I first came into professional baseball, there was a prevalent theory that weight lifting was not a positive thing for baseball players. This line of thought held that ballplayers did not need the overdeveloped upper body that was common among weight lifters, and, indeed, if they had such a physique they would be at a disadvantage.

Frankly, that theory is largely correct. Developing the wrong parts of your body for baseball can be less productive than doing no weight work at all.

Of course, the best thing to do is to work on the body so that its new strength and development are useful to you in baseball. That's what this program is designed to do.

I mention earlier that I had done a good deal of work and had been assisted in the development of the program by a number of other people. One of these is Mack Newton, who runs studios in Phoenix, Arizona. Newton himself is a fifth-degree black belt and a onetime world champion in Tae Kwon Do. He is also an expert on the most beneficial ways to prepare the body for exercise. He does some of the best stretching work I know of, and the first portion of this book is devoted to a stretching program for which I owe Mack a large debt.

Another man to whom I owe thanks for his time and effort in helping me formulate the program in the weight-lifting area is Gerry Robinson, operator of the ''Health for Life'' system in the Los Angeles area. He is always a source of information when I need it. Robinson appreciated the fundamental fact that baseball players are not bodybuilders in the traditional sense of that phrase. Rather, they are seeking to build their bodies for specific types of functions.

The way this book is structured is that the stretching portion is done first, since that is what happens in the normal course anyway. Never begin any exercise, game, or gym session without proper and sufficient warm-up and stretching.

There are certain things that I never let a ballplayer do. Before we begin to examine the program, let me set out a couple of them:

1. I never let a ballplayer begin a session without proper stretching.

2. I never let a ballplayer ''fight'' a weight. The key is to find the weight that works right for your body. Perfect form and technique are vital. If you are fighting to hold your balance on a lift, you run a high chance of injury and will accomplish little that is positive.

3. I actively discourage the use of steroids and other such drugs. They

may make muscular development come easier, but you pay for it later on. Whatever short-term gain there might be, it isn't worth the price your body will eventually have to pay. There is no room for steroids in this program or any other program for a serious athlete. Those drugs change the body's chemical balance, and any medical practitioner can give you plenty of reason why that is not a good idea.

4. I strongly urge that great caution be used with gym machines with which you are not thoroughly familiar. When you encounter a machine you haven't worked before, do a couple of light sets on it to get the feel of the machine. Know as much about the machine as you can and make sure that it is designed to help you achieve what you want to achieve.

We use many machines in the various gyms we use in the different American League cities. I make it my business to carefully check out the machines in each gym before I permit any of our players to use them. I will say, however, that the newer equipment coming on the market is generally better than what we used in the past simply because it is more adjustable to the individual needs of the user.

5. I never allow the players to compete with one another in the gym. In my opinion, this is a foolish practice for anybody. Weight lifting is not a competition except when a competitive weight-lifting event is being held. The purpose of being in the gym is to achieve certain things for your body, to improve your health and your performance. Competing with your buddy is not really the way to go unless you are professionals in the strength competitive areas. It creates a strong temptation to cheat on lifts, and it causes some people to do lifts that are not helpful. Obviously, it can also lead to inury, which is the last thing a ballplayer wants.

Now let's move on to the stretching program that we have developed for the team. There will first be a full-length program that we begin in off-season training. Then we will progress through the program as we generally taper it down to a maintenance-type program.

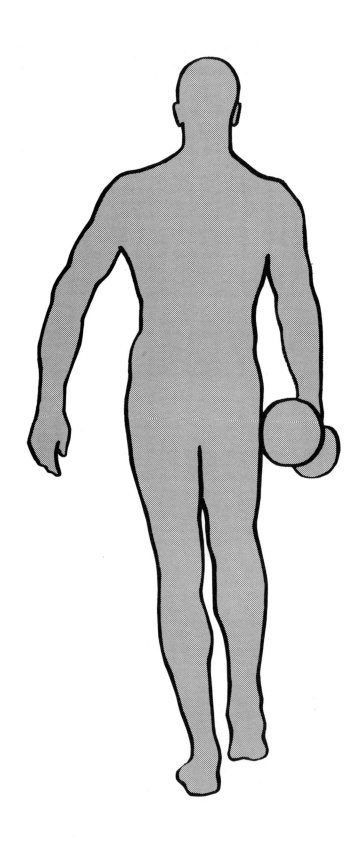

This program addresses thorough stretching for different parts of the body: torso, legs, arms, abdominal area, inner groin and quads, and back.

There are a few basic rules here. First, don't hurry your stretching. It is important to stretch the muscles and improve circulation. Stretching is not something that is delaying your getting to work; it is *part* of your work. Never stretch into pain or even into discomfort. Pain is a message from your body. If you are stretching into pain, stop. Don't bounce while stretching. This is a common practice, but it is counterproductive. It is important to maintain the breathing while stretching. This helps the muscles. Don't ever hold your breath while stretching. Always concentrate on the muscles being stretched. You can — and should — feel it happen. A lot of people like to stretch to music. This is fine if you think it helps. I do.

The Torso

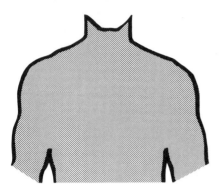

1 Begin by squeezing your body. Take a deep breath and hold it. Hold it for a five count (about five seconds). Then breathe and relax. While you are holding your breath, spread arms and legs. Spread the fingers. Tense the whole body. Think squeeze. Squeeze the chest, the shoulders, legs, calves, toes, neck. Squeeze each muscle group for a five count. Then breathe and relax, shaking the arms and legs out after each five seconds. Repeat this process for three sets, concentrating on squeezing different parts of the body.

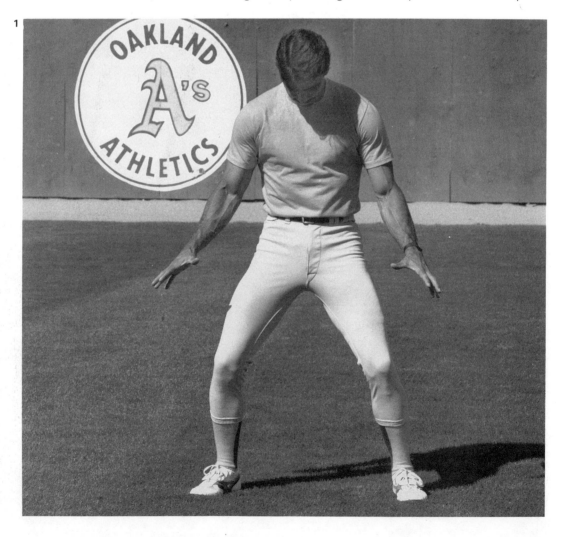

2 Now we will do a three-part stretch. Breathe during each one and don't hold it in.

2A Interlock your fingers over your head. Stretch upward, reaching for the sky. (Hold for 10 seconds.)

2B Same position, but this time twist to left (15 seconds).

2C Same position, but now twist to the right (15 seconds). Remember to breathe during each stretch.

2

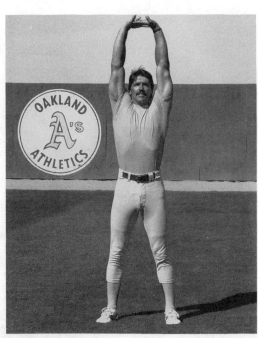

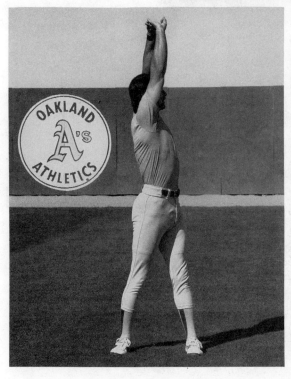

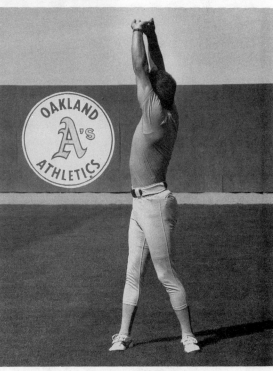

The Torso

Now place your hand on your hip. Start with the left hand on the left hip. **3A** Lean to the left (hold for 15 seconds), return upright, and remember to breathe during the stretch.

3A START

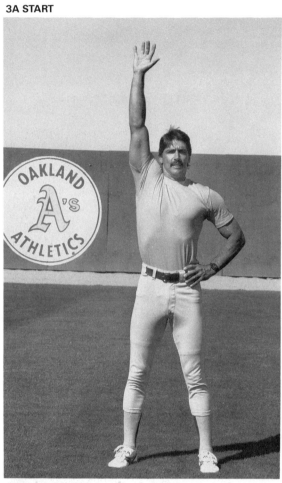

FINISH

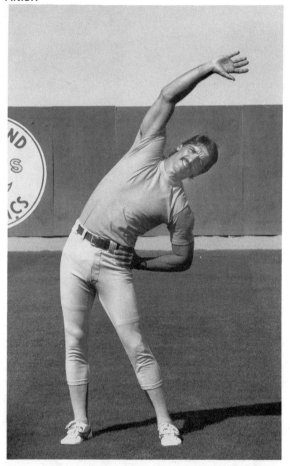

3B With the right hand on the right hip, lean to the right (15 seconds), return upright, and remember to breathe during the stretch.

FINISH

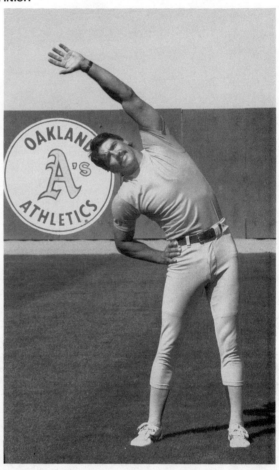

3B START

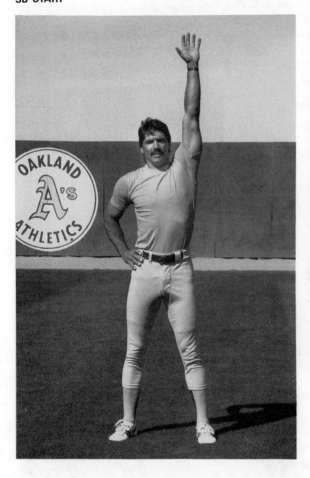

The Torso

4 Hold either forearm with your hand held behind your back, spread the legs, bend the knees, and then slowly lean back as far as you can (10 seconds) and return upright. Breathe.

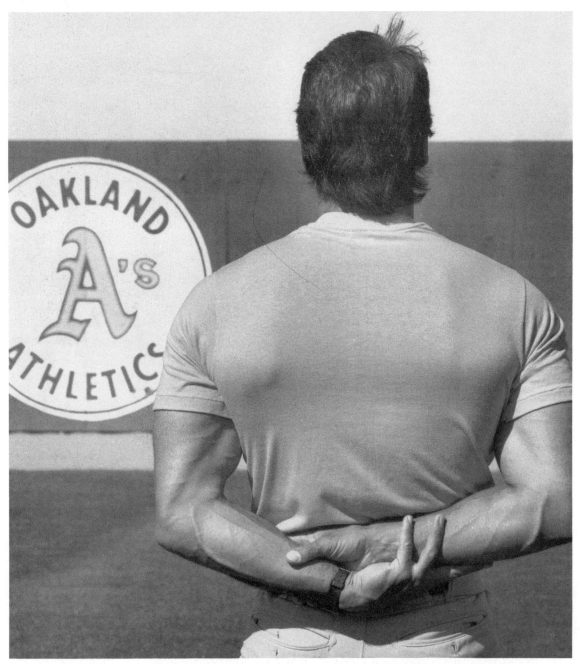

4 BACK VIEW START

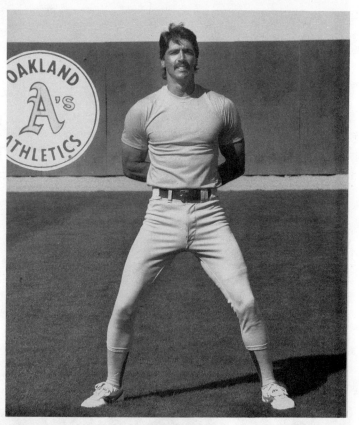

4 FRONTVIEW START

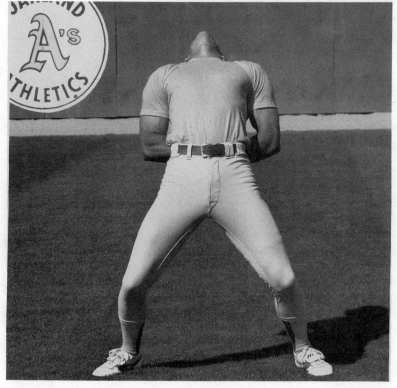

4 FINISH

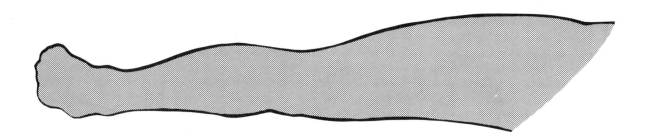

5 Keep your hands behind your back with legs spread and slowly lean forward. Arch your back with the chin up and hold (15 seconds). Your weight should be on the balls of your feet during this exercise.

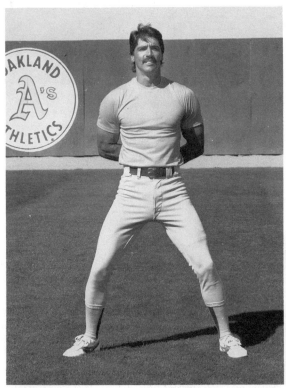

5 START

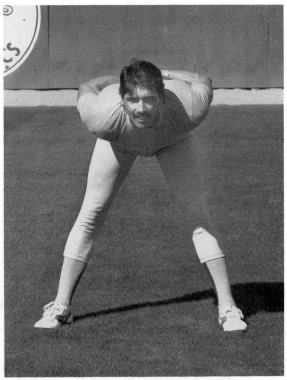

5 FINISH

6A Now move through a three-part sequence and, during each sequence, relax the shoulder and breathe. First, release your hands to the floor and hold (15 seconds).

6B Next, push up on the toes (10 seconds) and again relax the shoulders and breathe during the ten count.

6C Third, push up on the heels (10 seconds).

6A START

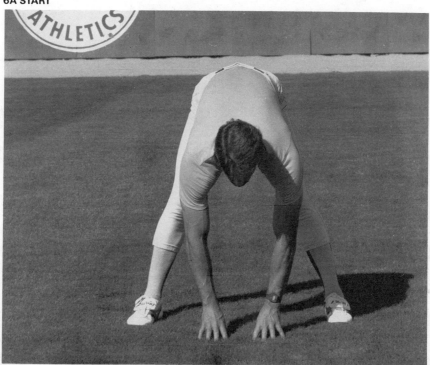

6B

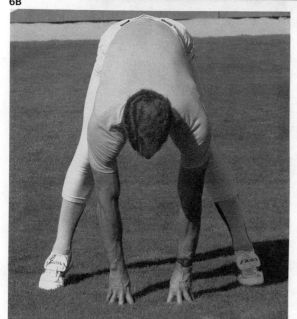

6C

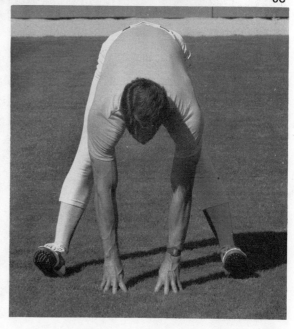

7A Now comes a four-part sequence in which you will "walk" your hands, as shown. First walk your hand to the left knee, keep your chin up, and hold (15 seconds).

7B Now walk your hand down to the ankle for a deeper stretch. Again, chin up and stomach to thigh (15 seconds) remembering to breathe.

7 START

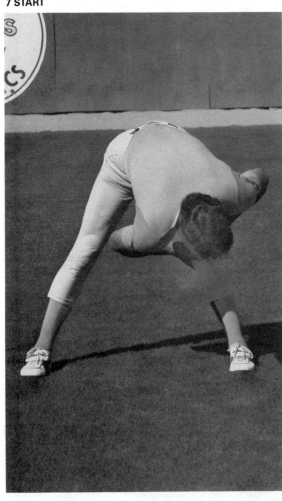

7B

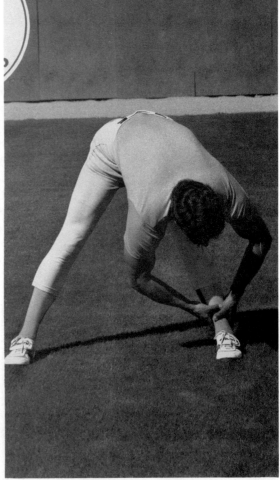

7C Now reverse the movement. Walk the hand across to the right side behind the knee (hold for 15 seconds).

7D Walk the hand down to the ankle on the right just as you did the left (15 seconds) and breathe.

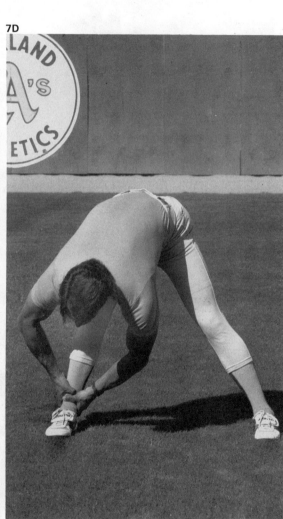

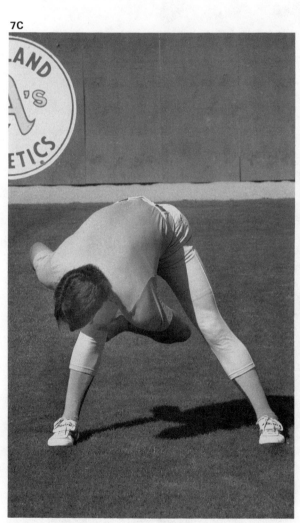

8 Walk the arms back to the midsection, walk the legs out wider, then just hang (15 seconds) and breathe. This is what I call the waterfall stretch, because you are just hanging like a waterfall.

8

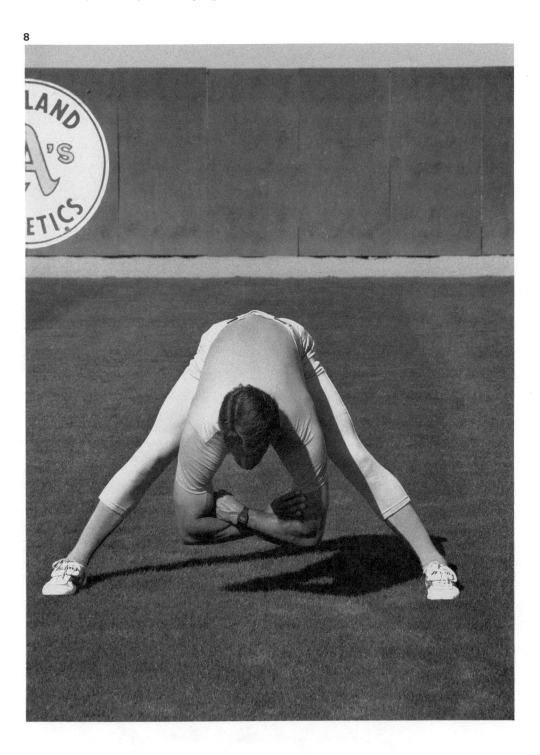

9 Now bring the feet a little closer together and squat into a spider stretch. Hold the chin up, arch your back and get the upper part of the legs parallel to the floor (15 seconds).

9

10 After you straighten out your legs, walk them together, cross your arms and again hang like a waterfall (15 seconds).

10A

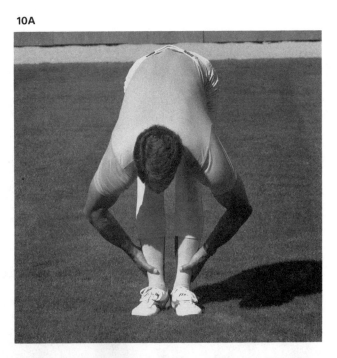

10B

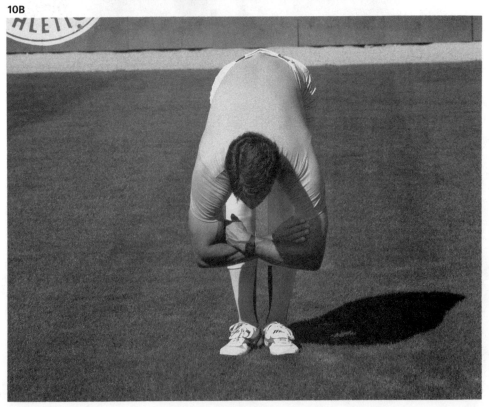

11 Bend the knees and stand upright.

11

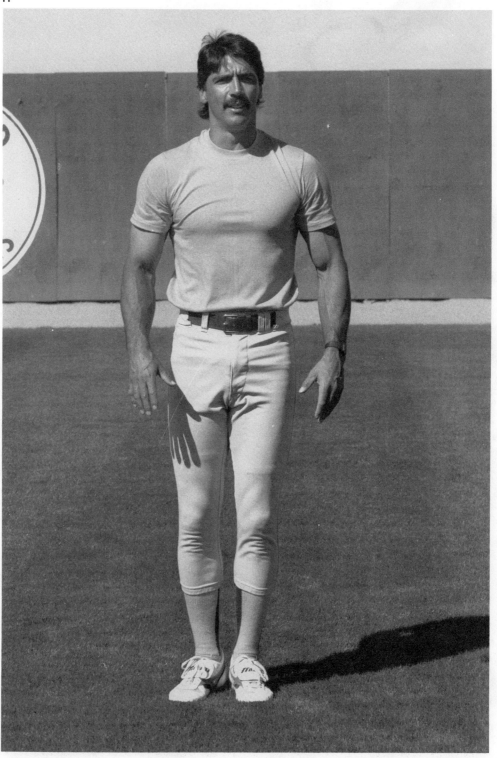

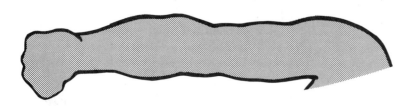

12 Relaxing your shoulders, pull into the stretch with your left elbow and right hand (15 seconds).

12B Then reverse, using the right elbow and left hand (15 seconds). Obviously, if you wish to do any of these alternate-side stretches opposite from the way they are shown, that's fine. You might be more comfortable starting with the right side rather than the left or vice versa. Go ahead.

12

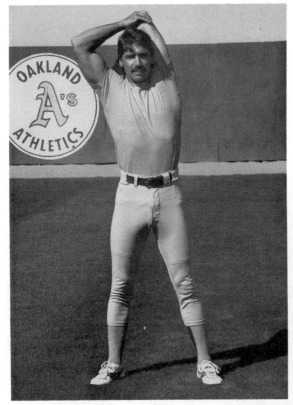

12B

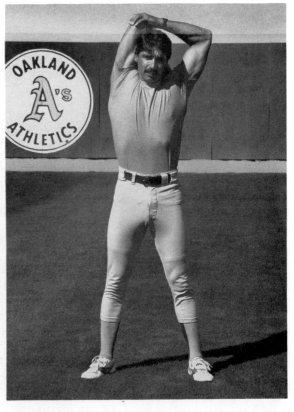

13A With your left arm across the front of your body parallel to the floor, the right hand pulls gently into the stretch (hold 15 seconds).

13B Take a deep breath, then exhale as you take the stretch further, ending with your chin over the shoulder (hold for 10 seconds).

13A

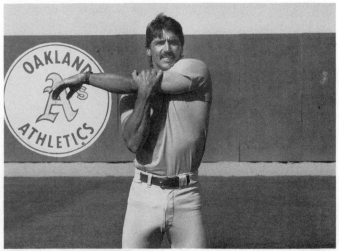

13B

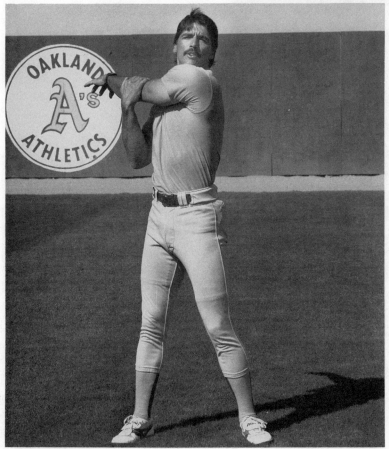

Arms

14A Now reverse the stretch. Right arm across the front, parallel to the floor and the left hand gently pulls into the stretch (15 seconds).

14B Take the deep breath, exhale, and take the stretch further to finish again with the chin over the shoulder (10 seconds).

14A

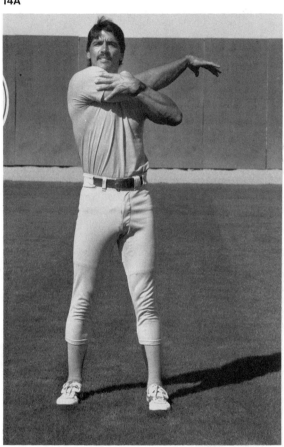

14B

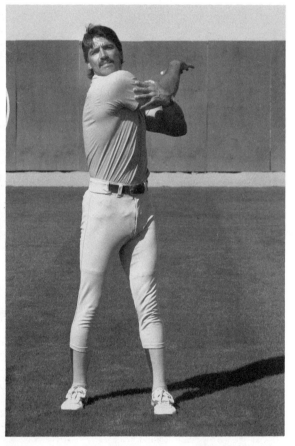

15 Here's a three-part warm-up that is done standing with a slight spread of the legs and arms extended straight out to your sides with palms downward. All of these movements are done at a medium speed.

15A Start making small forward circles and keep count until you have done 25 circles.

15B Now make the circles a little larger and do 25 more.

15C Make the circles larger yet and do 25 more.

After you have done the last 25 circles, stop and shake the arms out.

15A

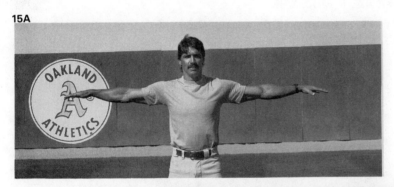

15B

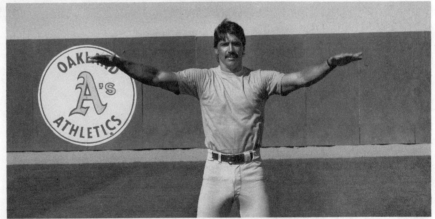

15C

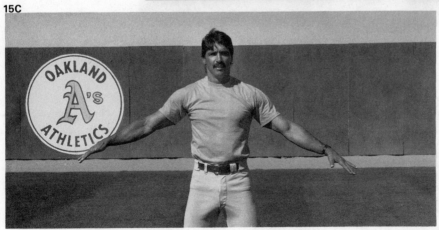

16 Now we're going to do the same thing in reverse. Assume the same position: stand with a slight spread of the legs and arms extended straight out with palms facing upward.

16A Again using a medium speed, make 25 small circles, only this time do them backward.

16B Now make 25 circles backward, just slightly larger.

16C To finish, make 25 more circles backward, a little bigger than the ones before. Again, this is not a race against the clock. Do all the movements at medium speed to maximize the benefit.

When you finish your last 25 circles, stop and shake the arms out again.

16A

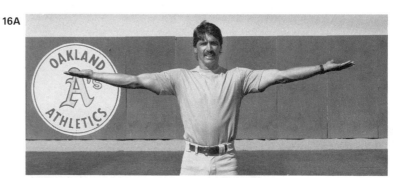

16B

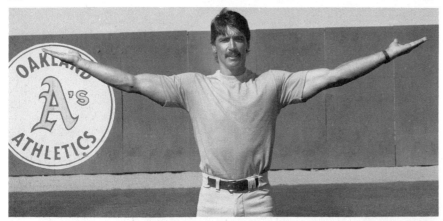

16C

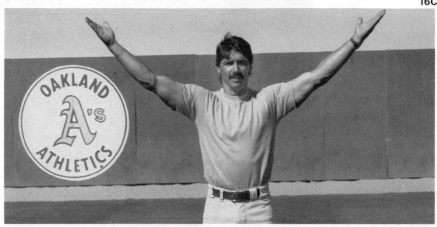

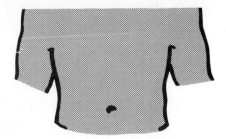

17 With fingers laced together behind your head, bend your knees and keep your feet flat on the floor. Keep your lower back flat on the floor, concentrate on the stomach doing the lifting, and lift the shoulder off the floor. (Hold for 30 seconds.) Lower and repeat for a second set. Do not hold your breath during this stretch. Breathe normally.

During the course of the stretching exercises and the weight workouts that follow, I will sometimes use the word *think* when in the midst of a set to suggest that you should be focusing your concentration on a certain part of the body or trying to achieve a certain state of mind with respect to a set. It is important that you have a clear mind when you are doing any type of workout in order to achieve the most that the set has to offer. There is, of course, a certain relaxing quality to this. But the fundamental here is that you must concentrate on what the set is designed to achieve. One of the examples of this is the 6-inch leg raises that follow.

17A

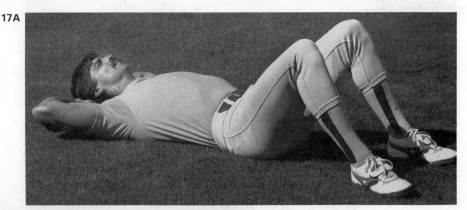

17B

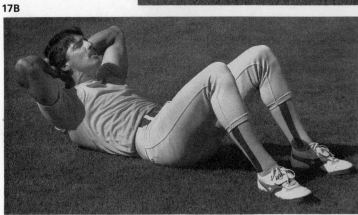

18 With arms straight, palms flat on the floor tucked just under the sides of the buttocks, lift your shoulders just off the floor and relax your body. Raise your feet about 16 inches off the floor. Now you are ready to begin. Exhale and shrink the stomach. Think the navel to the spine, compress the stomach. This should cause the feet to elevate about 6 or less inches (no higher) without having to use your legs to lift the feet. As you breathe in, your feet should lower back to about 16 inches off the floor. Exhale again and they will raise up again. Repeat this inhaling and exhaling for 25 repetitions at a medium speed. By medium speed, I mean about one rep per second. After 25 reps, take a 15-second rest and then repeat the process for another 20 reps. At first, you may not be able to do 20 reps in the second cycle. If that is the case, do as many as you can.

After you have done the second sequence of leg raises, take a 15-second rest and move on immediately to the abdominal crunches.

18 START

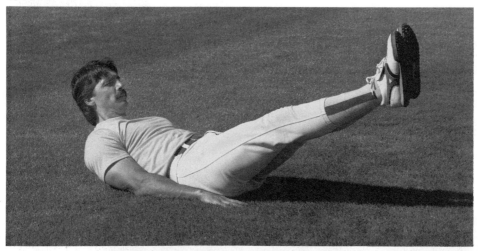

18 FINISH

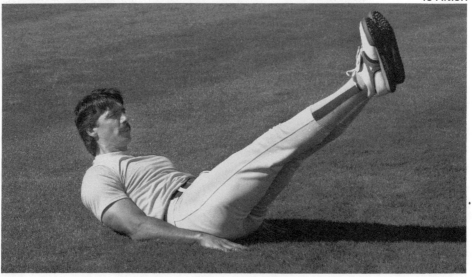

19 Interlock your fingers behind the head and bend the knees with the feet flat. Again, concentrate on the stomach doing the lifting and lift the shoulders off the floor. Pause at the top and then lower the shoulders. Repeat for 25 reps at a slow pace. A slow pace is a rate of 1 for every 2 seconds. Keep the elbows flared out.

    Without taking a rest, move directly on to the quarter sit-up.

19

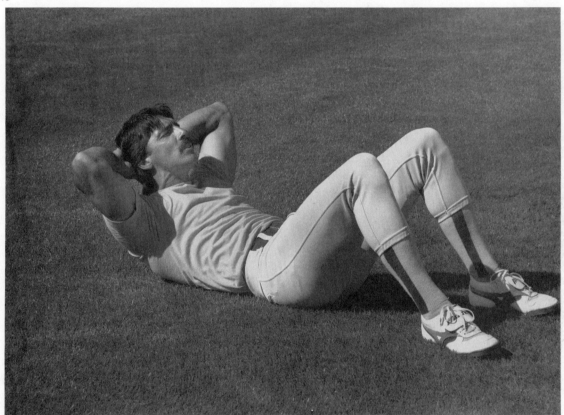

Abdominal Work

20 With fingers still interlocked behind the head, bring the legs up, crossing at the ankles with the quads straight up. Concentrating on using the abdominals only, lift the shoulders off the floor at a fast speed — that is, about 2 per second. Do as many as possible. If you are using the abdominals properly, you should not be able to do more than 10 to 15 reps. This is designed to work the upper abdominal muscles. Once you have completed as many as you can, take a 20-second rest.

20 START

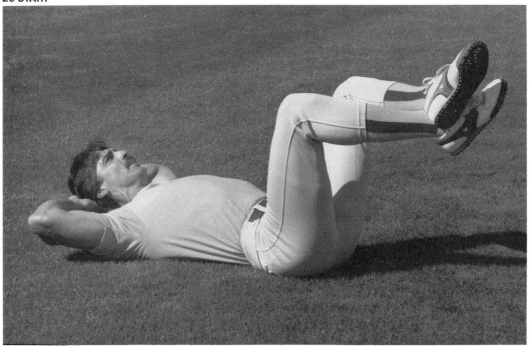

20 FINISH

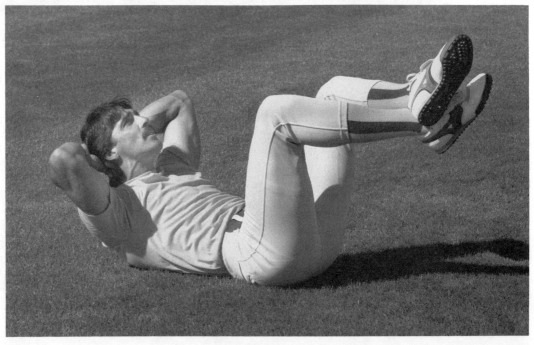

21 Then, lying flat on your back with arms out to the sides and palms flat down, raise your legs straight up. Lower your legs to the right until they are approximately 6 inches off the floor, then raise them back up. Then lower your legs to the left side. Repeat this for 10 reps each way. This is a good exercise for the obliques.

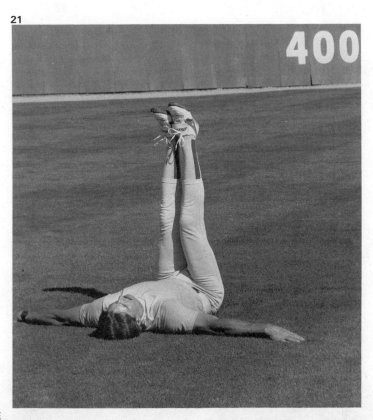

21

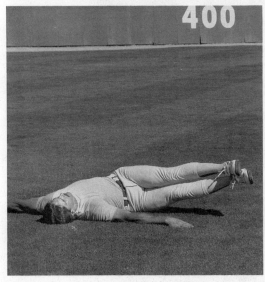

21 RIGHT SIDE

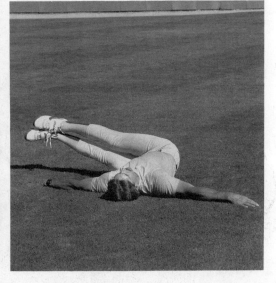

21 LEFT SIDE

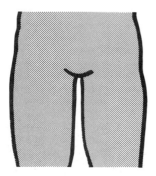

22 Now get down on your knees with your instep flat on the ground and place your hands on your heels. Lie back and push out on the hips. Breathe (10 seconds).

22

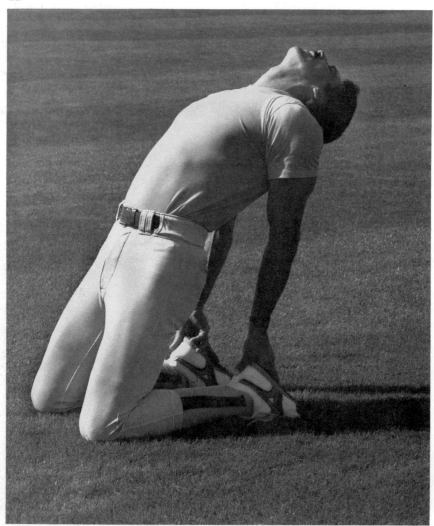

23 With your toes together, spread your legs as much as possible.
23A Lower your hips and feel the stretch (hold 10 seconds).
23B Come back off the stretch, rounding your back as you do so, and you can feel the comfort in this stretch (15 seconds).

23

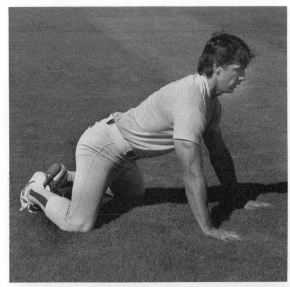

23A

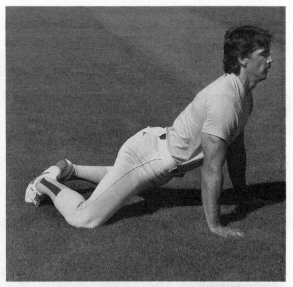

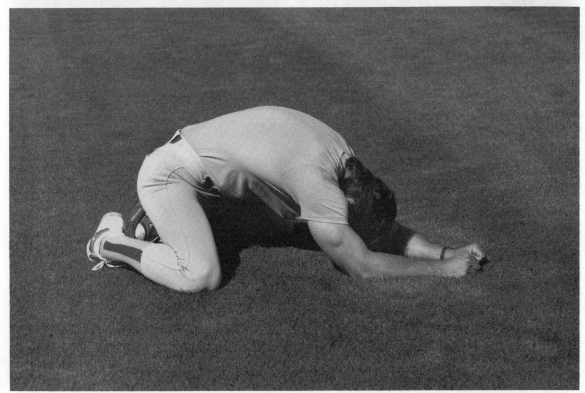

23B

24 Now, lying straight out on your stomach, pointing the fingers straight out, lift up the hands and the feet as high as possible. Breathe (10 seconds).
24A Again come back into this comfortable stretch, this time for 15 seconds.

24

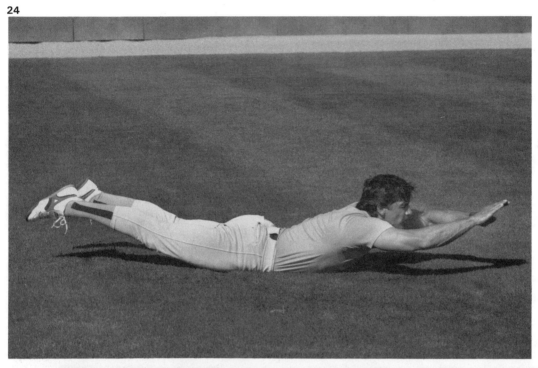

24A

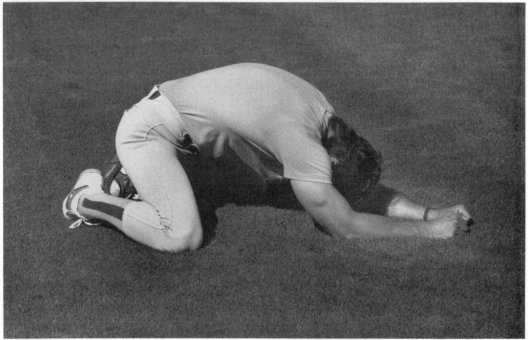

Now we're going into a 4-point groin stretch.

25 Place the right leg ahead of the left with the left knee about 1 inch off the floor and the front leg at a 45-degree angle. Lower the hips and hold for 15 seconds.

25A With the back knee on the floor and the instep flat, reach with the right hand under the leg with the palm on the instep. Rest your left elbow on the floor if you can, or as far as you can go, and feel the stretch (15 seconds).

25

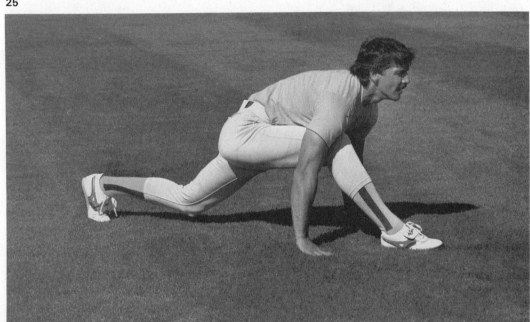

25A

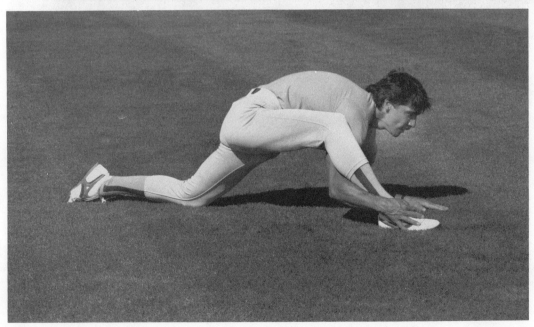

Inner Groin and Quads

25B Then reach back with the right hand to the left foot. Pull the foot to the buttocks, then lean forward into the stretch (15 seconds).

25C Now lean back, placing the hands on the hips, pushing the hips forward as you lean back (10 seconds).

25B

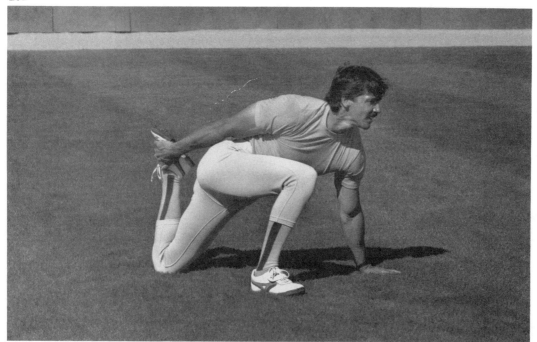

25C

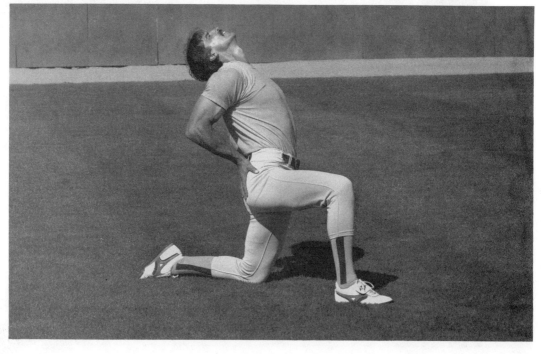

Now we're going to do this whole sequence in reverse. Again, you may do these sequences either way. I have done them in the order in which I prefer them.

26 This time, put the left leg forward with the back knee about 1 inch off the floor, the front leg at a 45-degree angle. Lower the hips and hold for 15 seconds.

26A With the back knee on the ground and the instep flat, reach with the left hand under the leg with the palm on the instep. Rest your right elbow on the floor (15 seconds).

26

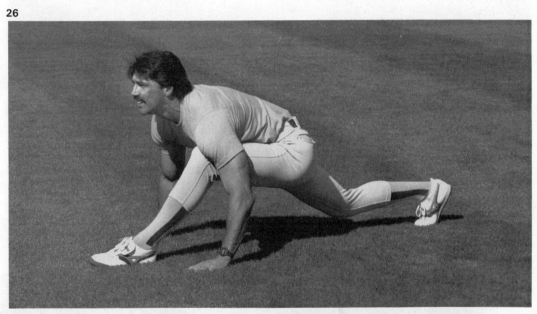

26A

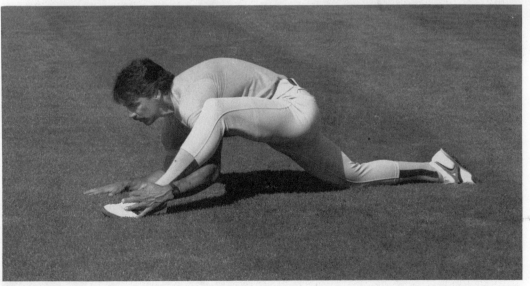

Inner Groin and Quads

26B Reach back with the left hand to the right foot. Pull the foot to the buttocks and then lean forward into the stretch (15 seconds).
26C Lean back, place the hands on the hips and push the hips forward as you lean back (10 seconds).

26B

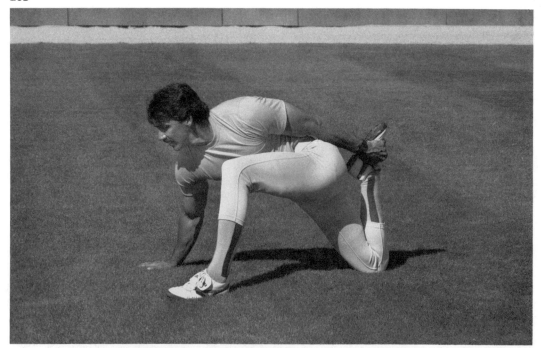

26C

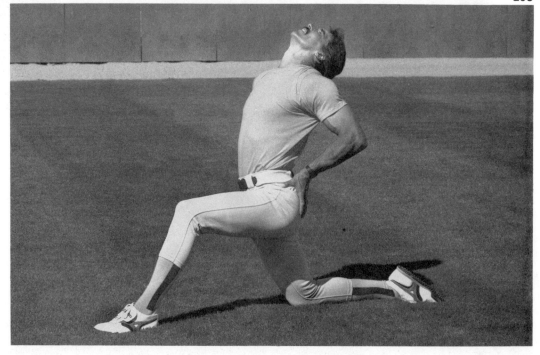

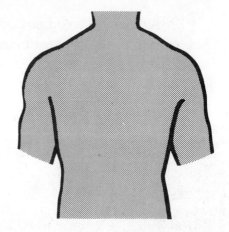

27A Lying flat on your back with your hands out to your sides, put the left leg over the right and feel the stretch (15 seconds).
27B For a deeper stretch, reach with the left hand and pull down on the left knee. Breathe (15 seconds).

27A

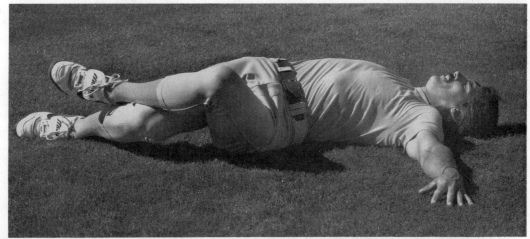

27 B

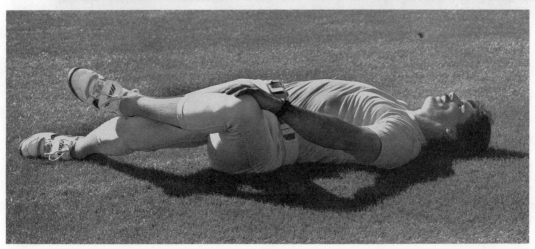

Back

28A Lying on your back with your hands out to your side, put the right leg over the left. Feel the stretch (15 seconds).
28B Reach up with the right hand and pull down on the right knee for the deeper stretch (15 seconds) and breathe.

28A

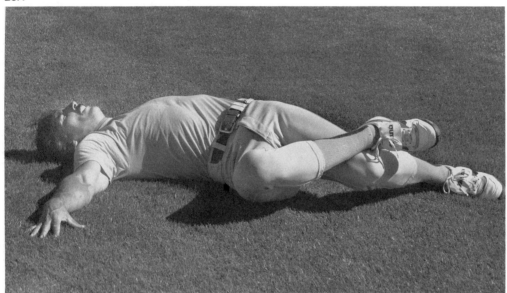

28 B

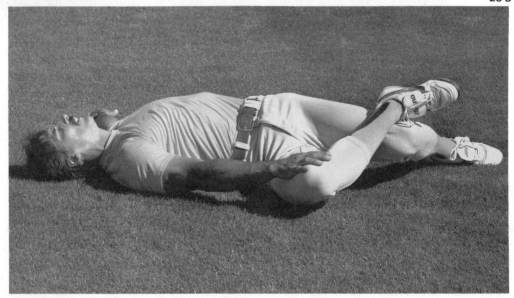

29A Sitting up with the right leg crossed over the left, twist to your right with the left arm pushing against the outside of your right leg. Feel the stretch and breathe (15 seconds).

29B Twisting to your left, with the right arm on the inside of the right leg, feel the stretch and breathe (15 seconds).

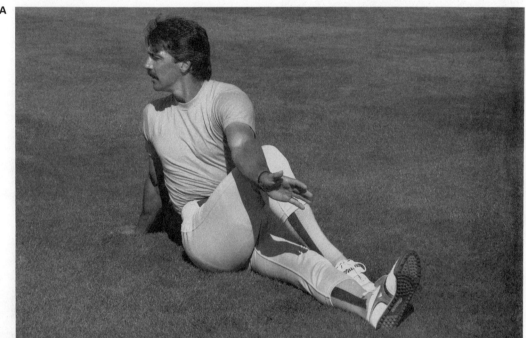

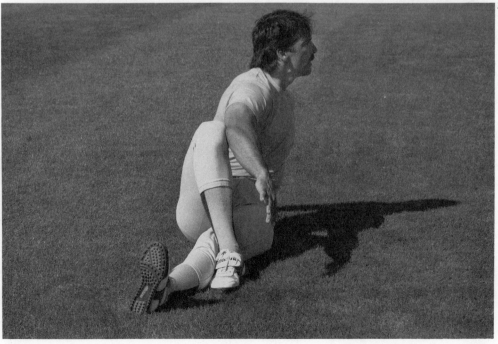

Back

30A Sitting up with the left leg over the right, twist to your left with the right arm pushing against the outside of the left leg. Feel the stretch and breathe (15 seconds).

30B Twisting to your right, right arm pushing on the inside of the right leg, feel the stretch and breathe (15 seconds).

30A

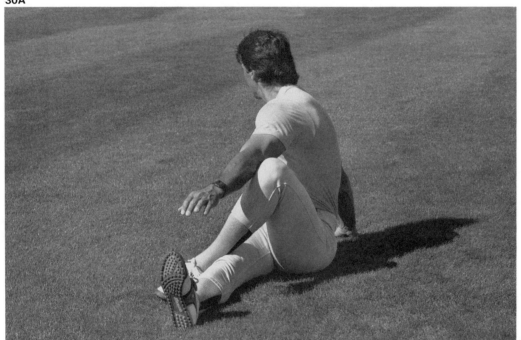

30 B

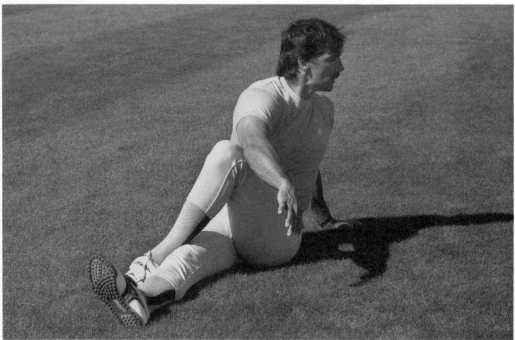

31 Now stand straight up with hands straight up. Start rotating the upper body to each side, exhaling as you do. Keep the feet pointed straight ahead. Start easy and feel the back loosen up with each rotation. You can do 50 rotations in each direction, but don't push it.

31

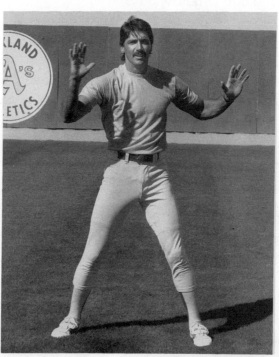

31 TO LEFT

31 TO RIGHT

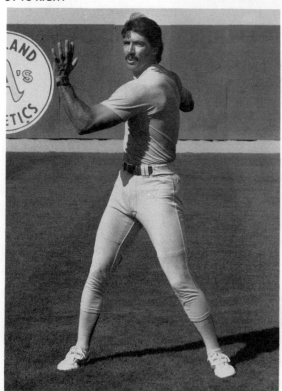

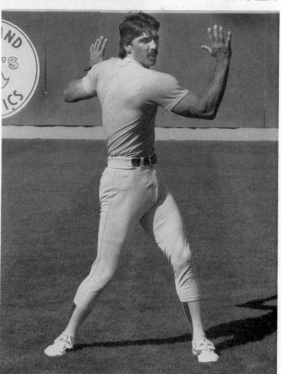

32 To finish the back stretches, sit with legs crossed, relax, and take a few deep breaths.

This stretching program was developed originally for ballplayers and is designed to improve muscle tone and circulation as well as to get players loose before a game or before a workout.

However, this program is valuable for anyone at any time. A good stretch is important before any kind of physical activity. You don't have to be a major-league ballplayer to learn to take care of your body. Obviously, the better care you take of your body, the better it will work for you. You will feel fitter and healthier. This can improve your performance in recreational sports or at the office.

32

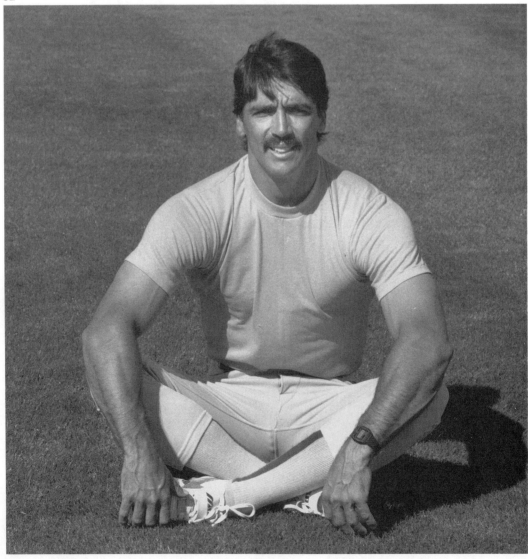

Much of what I have to say about weight training I have acquired through working with Dave McKay since I joined the Oakland Athletics. But I have always had an interest in weight training.

However, the following program is one specifically designed for use by ballplayers, and it is the best one I know of in or out of the major leagues for that purpose. Certainly from the standpoint of the improvement in performance by ballplayers who have used the program, the results speak for themselves.

Dave and I do want to stress a few basic points.

1. Find a safe weight to start your work. A guide in this area is to find a weight you can bench press to fatigue at a rate of about 8 to 10 repetitions for upper body and more repetitions for the lower body.

2. A safe weight is a comfortable weight. It is never beneficial to lift more than you are comfortable with; because to do so you will have to leave perfect form and technique.

3. Perfect form and technique are essential elements of any successful weight-training program. Without perfect form and technique, you cannot realize the entire value of any program. Many professionals have analyzed weights for many years to develop the best form for their use. There is a reason for this. Understand that and you can begin to maximize the value of weight training.

4. Always use a spotter on heavy routines such as a bench press or military press. A partner can help you get the last two or three lifts to perfect form, which gives you the most benefit from the work.

5. Always use a belt on any upright lift.

6. Pace yourself when you lift. Between lifts, I strive for a rhythm of not less than 30 seconds or more than 45 seconds rest between lift. But if your body tells you it needs more time to rest, take that time. You're not trying to punish your body, you're trying to develop it to maximum efficiency and productivity.

One of the more foolish things that lifters do is cheat on a lift. This usually happens because they are engaged in a competition with somebody else in the gym. Don't let your ego get in the way of a good work with your weight-training program. You should have a purpose for your work, and that purpose is what you are striving for. Don't waste your time and get sidetracked.

We are fortunate in that we have Dave to establish some basic discipline for what we are doing. But whether you have somebody like him or not, try not to lose sight of your goals in the gym. If you do, you will just be wasting time and probably money.

I would also like to reemphasize that this program is not designed to make you look good at the beach. If that is your goal, that's okay. But it isn't the purpose behind this program. This program is specifically for those who want to improve the potential of their body for baseball.

I have found that, if you follow it correctly, it is a program that can be of great help. I believe that it can help anyone who is in the majors improve their performance. It can also help any ballplayer who is not in the majors improve their performance as well.

This program will not make you a major-league baseball player all by itself. Playing baseball is hard work and requires a wide range of skills and disciplines. But it will certainly help.

We will go through all of the basic lifts and routines that we use and then we will follow with several sample programs. These are basically the programs we use on the ballclub. Some of them are good for off-season work, some of them are best for spring training, and some of them are for in-season.

We have labeled them as off-season, spring training, and in-season programs. But we have also set them up on a rotation for a certain number of days. Thus, if you are not a pro ballplayer, you may be able to pick a program that works well for you and vary it from time to time with another longer or shorter program.

That is a worthwhile thought. Vary your programs some and, above all, make sure that you are not overdoing it. Many lifters have the idea that they should do more all the time. That is not necessarily the case. A muscle has only a hundred percent to give, as Dave is fond of saying, and it can't give you any more than that.

There are times when the best thing you can do for your body is give it an easy day or a complete day off. Keep this in mind.

One of the tricks here is to communicate with your body and listen to what it is telling you. Your body has many ways of giving feedback. Pain. Fatigue. These are information signs from your body. Don't ignore them.

Also, don't rush into a day's work. Always do a thorough stretch before you even think of lifting or hitting a machine. Make sure you are warmed up and loose.

To begin the weight-training program, we use one of the best and oldest exercises in the book — the push-up.

1 Push-ups should be done with hands a little wider than shoulder width. Keep the body rigid and the face down. Lower your body until the chest slightly touches the floor and then go back up. This is a nice, easy warm-up before starting light bench work. A tip: breathe in deeply through the nose when going down and blow out through the mouth when pushing up.

1 START

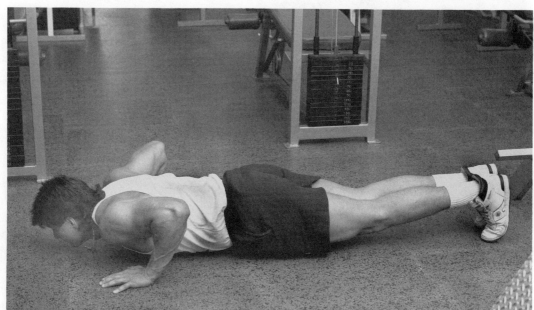

1 FINISH

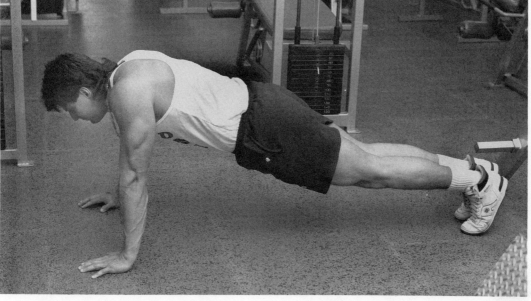

Proper Grip

2 Proper grip on the bars is important. Avoid gripping the bar too deep in the hands toward the fingers, because this will tend to bend the wrist back. Keep the bar resting on the heel of the hands with the wrist locked in a straight-up, pistonlike position.

2 RIGHT WAY

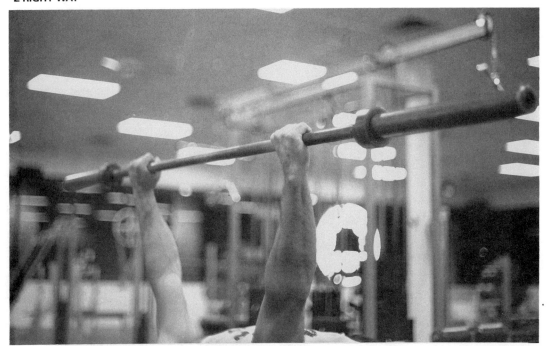

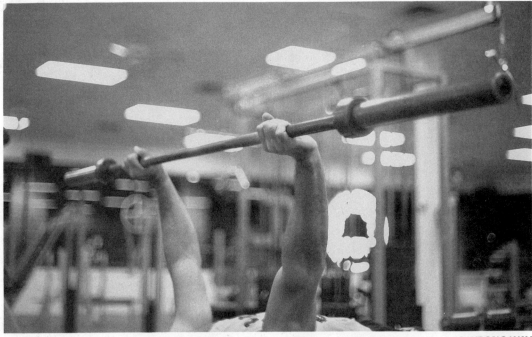

2 WRONG WAY

3 This is the basic bench press supine (flat) barbell lift for the chest. It works mainly with the middle pectoral (chest) muscles. Arms should be slightly angled out. If the grip is too close, it puts too much emphasis on the triceps; if the grip is too wide apart, it puts too much stress on the shoulders. As I am doing here, keep the lower back flat on the bench, slowly lowering the bar down to just above the sternum. Push up on an angle that takes the bar directly above the chin. At the peak of the lift, the shoulders should come off the bench. Avoid bouncing the bar off the chest. And remember the proper breathing technique: inhale as you lower the weight, blow out as you push it up. Putting your feet up on the bench will help to keep your back flat against the bench, especially for those of us who have a tendency to use too much leg and arch the back during the lift.

3 START

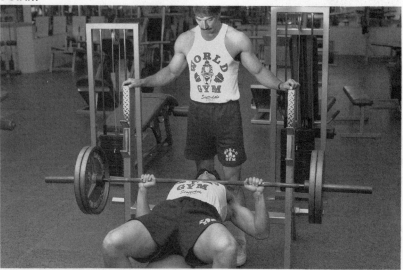

3 FINISH

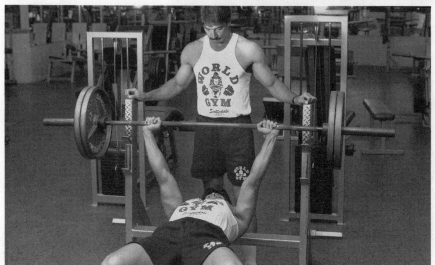

Bench Press Incline Barbell

4 This works primarily on the upper chest (pectorals). It is much the same as the supine bench press except that the bar will be lowered to the upper chest and will be pushed straight up instead of angled back. Set the bench on a steep angle and keep your back flat on the bench, or this lift becomes too much like the supine press. Again, bear in mind the proper breathing technique: inhale through the nose while lowering the bar and blow out through the mouth when pushing it up.

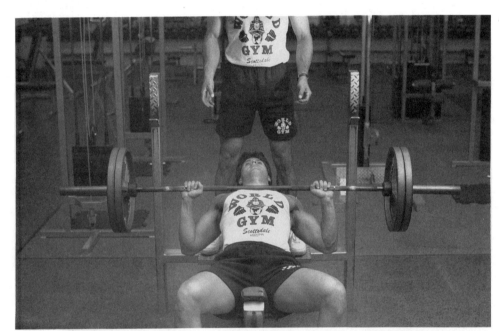

4 START

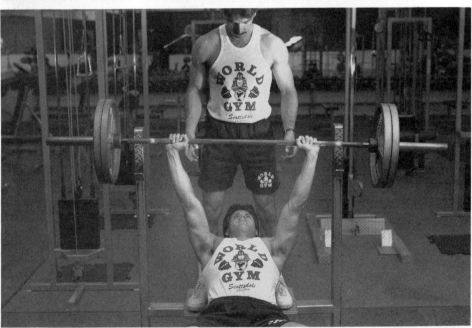

4 FINISH

5 Here is the lift for the lower chest. It is the same as the previous bench work except that you lower the bar to the middle of the chest, pushing straight up.

5 START

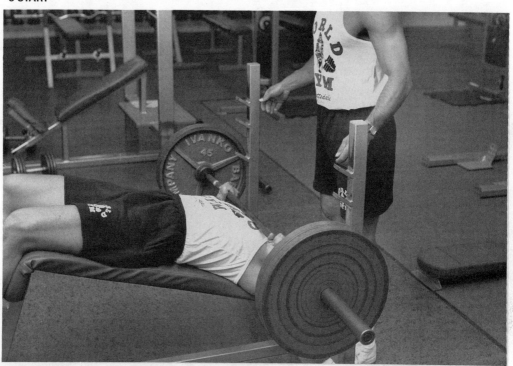

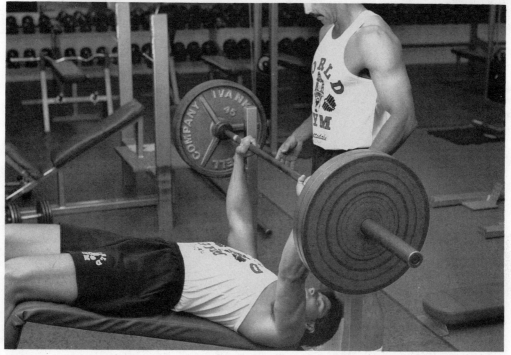

5 FINISH

Bench Press (Supine) Dumbbells

6A To exercise the middle pectorals, lower the dumbbells to the sides of the upper chest.

6A START

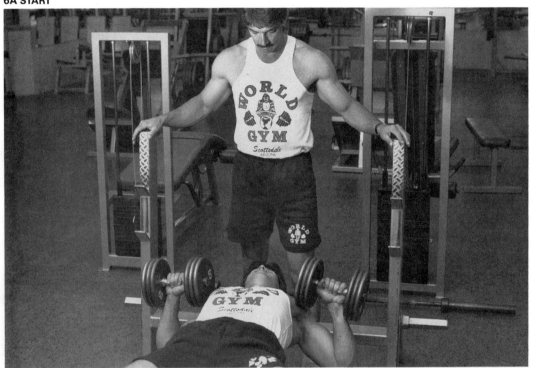

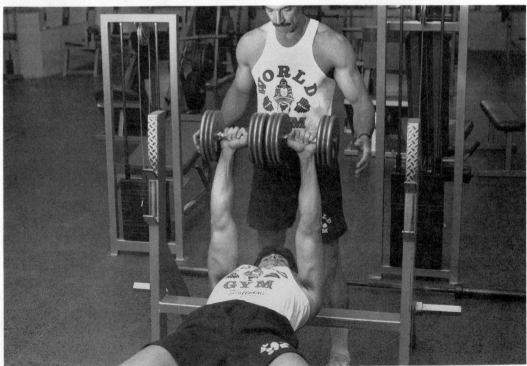

6A FINISH

6B Here we work the upper pectorals by lowering the dumbbells to the sides of the shoulders.

6B

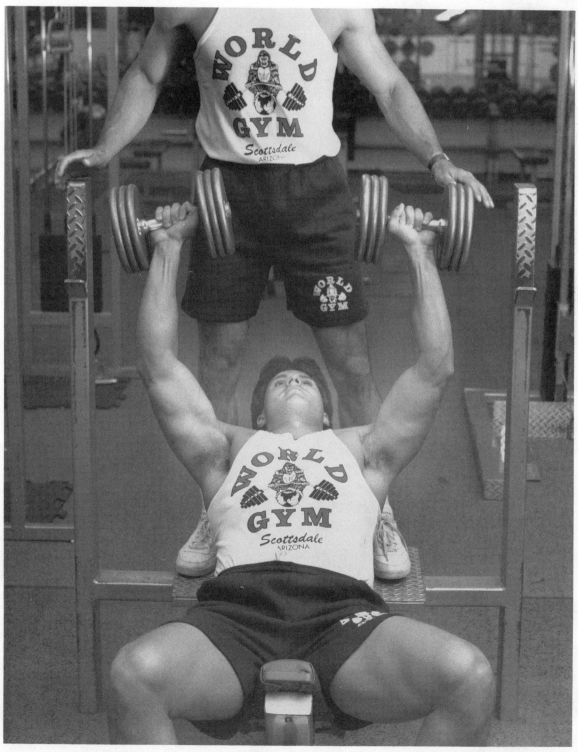

Bench Press (Incline) Dumbbells

6B START

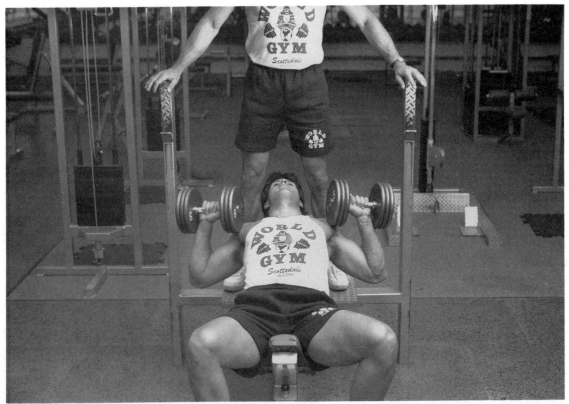

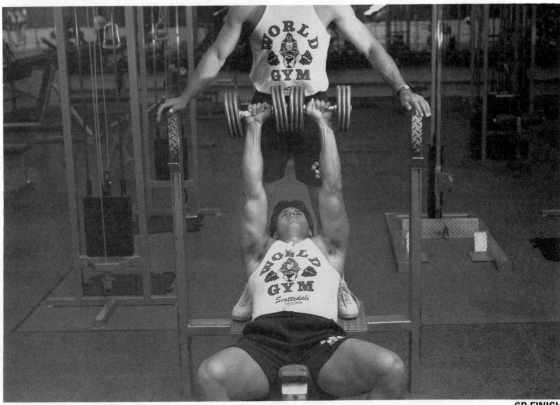

6B FINISH

6C Now we are working the lower pectorals by lowering the dumbbells to the sides of the lower chest. Each of these lifts is similar to the bench work with the barbells except that you hold the dumbbells parallel to each other. As you push upward, you bring the dumbbells lightly together on a slightly curved angle. The weights should end up almost touching. Avoid the straight line up or in. Lift the shoulders off the bench and lower back to the starting position feeling a comfortable stretch in the shoulders and the chest.

6C START

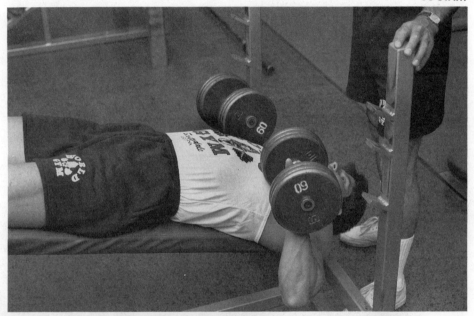

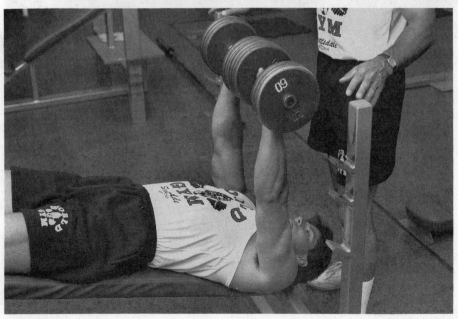

6C FINISH

Supine Dumbbell Flys

7 This works for the middle chest (middle pectorals). Hold the dumbbells above the chest with a comfortable bend in the elbows. Lower dumbbells off to the sides, keeping the elbows locked. Do not lower the dumbbells with the arms straight, because this places too much stress on the shoulders. Try to visualize doing these lifts with an imaginary barrel on your chest. Bring the dumbbells up and around this imaginary barrel to where they touch or almost touch. At the bottom of the lift, feel the stretch across the chest, pull the pecs together, and bring the dumbbells up. Throughout this exercise, think chest.

7 START

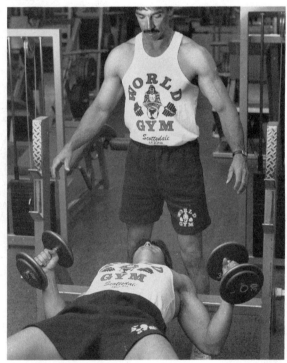

7 FINISH

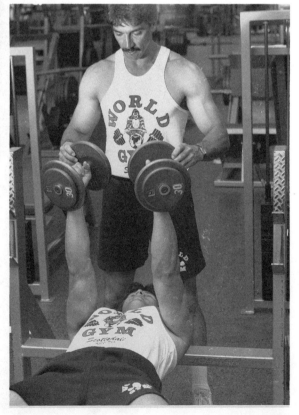

8 This is mainly for working the upper chest, and is basically the same as the supine dumbbell lifts except the starting position is slightly different since you are lowering the dumbbells to the side of the shoulders.

8 FINISH

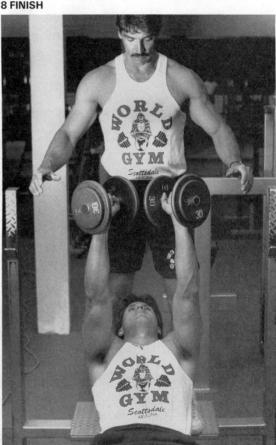

8 START

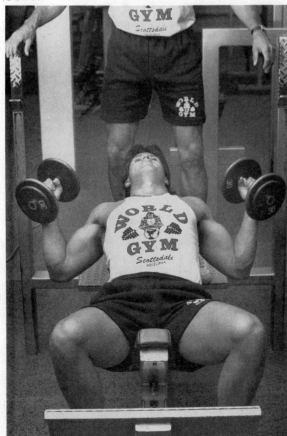

Cross-Body Cable Pulls

9 This is an effect for the middle and lower chest area, that section of the pectorals along the sternum. Stand straight up with arms fully extended and a slight bend in the elbows. As you begin to pull the grips together in a downward motion, your body should at the same time start to hunch over. Bring the grips together with the palms facing each other. Your arms should be pointing almost straight down. A slight bend in the elbows takes the stress off the shoulders. Raise and repeat. With each rep, maintain your breathing technique: breathe in as you come set and blow out into the lift as you lower.

9 START

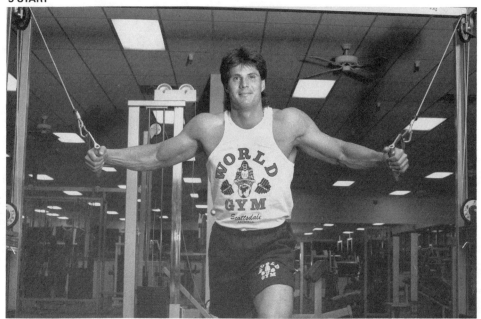

9 FINISH

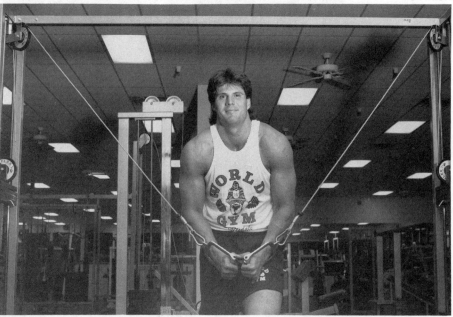

10 This routine works mainly the shoulders (the anterior and lateral deltoids). Use a weight belt to stabilize the lower back. Sit on a bench with a back support. As you can see from my position, it is important to concentrate on the back being flat against the back of the seat and avoid arching the back. You want a slightly wider grip here to avoid too much tricep involvement. Raise the bar directly over head, arms extended. Lower the bar behind the head until it just slightly touches the thicker upper back muscles just below the neck. Keep the elbows facing out in opposite directions. Do not overstrain when pushing up on the weight. This is a lift in which you should use a spotter. It is very important here to employ perfect form and technique as well as good breathing.

10 START

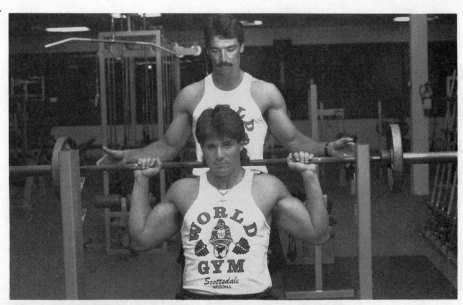

10 FINISH

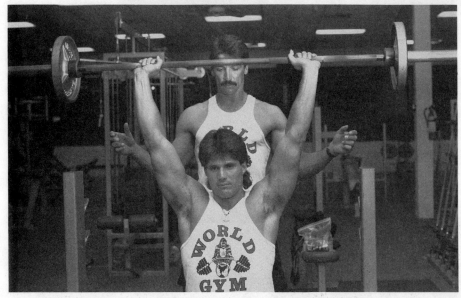

Seated Alternate Dumbbell Press

11 This works mainly for the shoulder (anterior and lateral deltoids). Use the same basic position as the military press, only the dumbbells will begin resting in line at the side of the shoulders, palms facing forward. Alternating from one side to the other, push one side up, the dumbbell peaking directly above the shoulder. Lower it back to the ready position and then raise the other side. Breathe in when coming down, and out when pushing up. It is a very good idea to use a belt when doing these lifts.

11 START

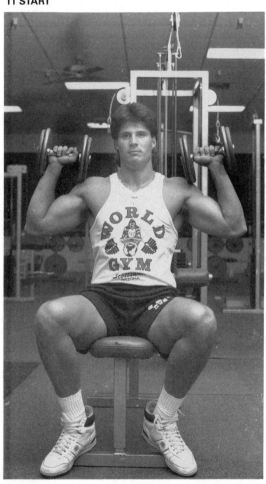

11 FINISH

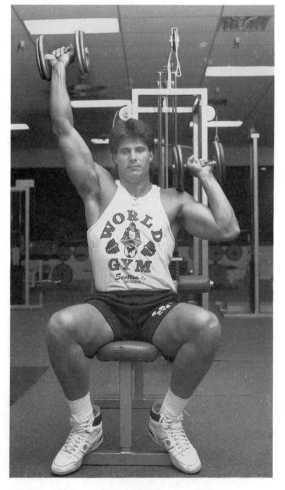

11 FINISH

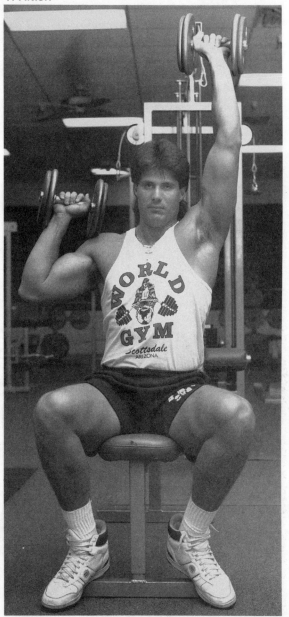

11 START

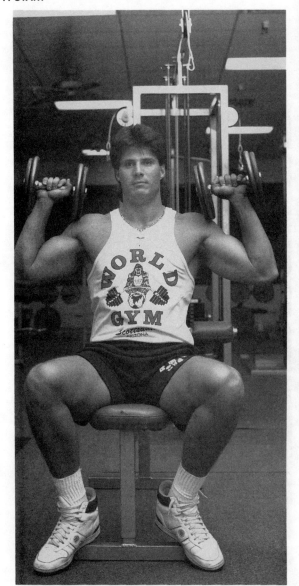

Upright Rows (Bar or Cables)

12 This is work for the shoulders (anterior and lateral deltoids). The grip here has the hands very close to touching. Pull the bar up to shoulder level. Keep the bar close to the body. Pause at the top of the lift and then lower. If the bar is held away from the body, it will work the front part of the shoulders only. A belt is recommended during this lift, and the lift should be done with a slight bend in the knees. Breathe in when going down, and out as you push the weight upward. When lifting the weight, force the elbows up high.

12 START

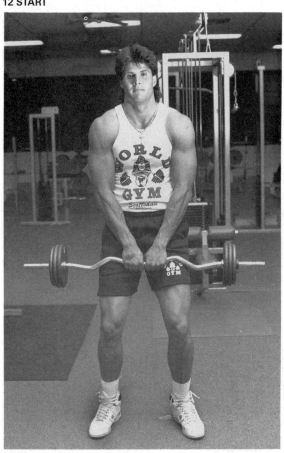

12 FINISH

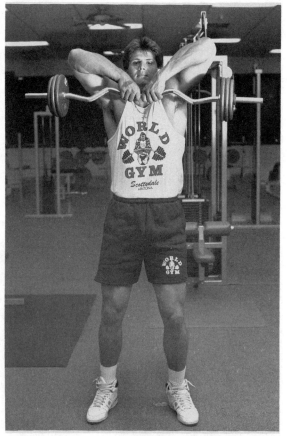

13 This is work for the lateral deltoids or the side deltoids (shoulders). Holding light dumbbells at your side (with a slight bend in the elbows to take the stress off the shoulders), raise the dumbbells to shoulder height, pause, and lower. During the lifts, your palms should begin facing each other and end facing down. A tip: If you can't pause at the top of the lift, you are using too much weight. Again, breathe in as you lower the dumbbells and blow out as you lift.

13 START

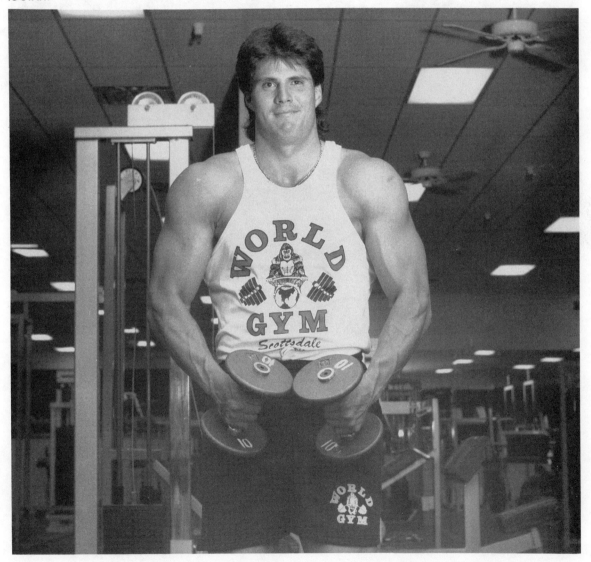

Lateral or Side Dumbbell Raises (Double-Arm)

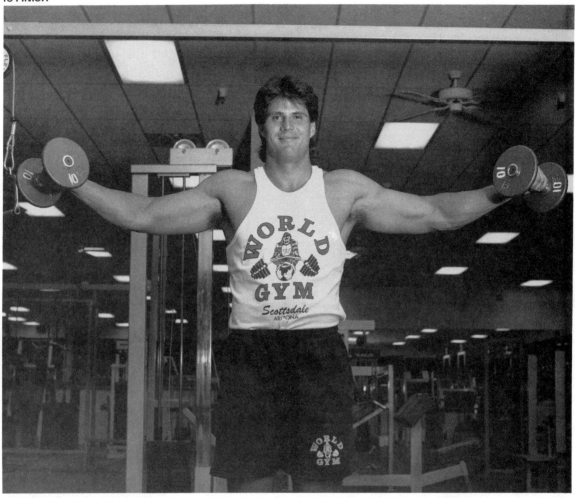

74

Anterior (Front) Dumbbell Raises (Double-Arm)

14 This routine works mainly for the front deltoids or anterior deltoids of the shoulder. Holding light dumbbells in front of you, bend the elbows slightly and raise the dumbbells to shoulder height, pause, and lower. Again, the palms should begin facing you and finish with the palms facing down.

14 START

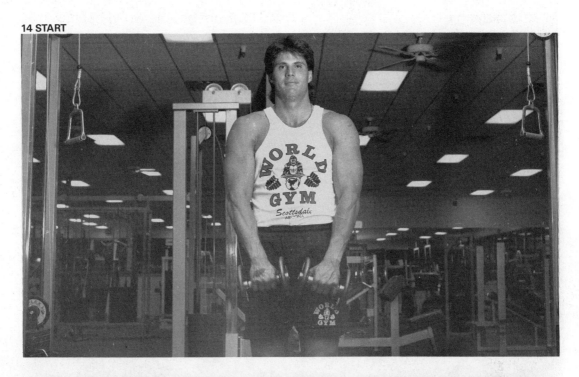

14 FINISH

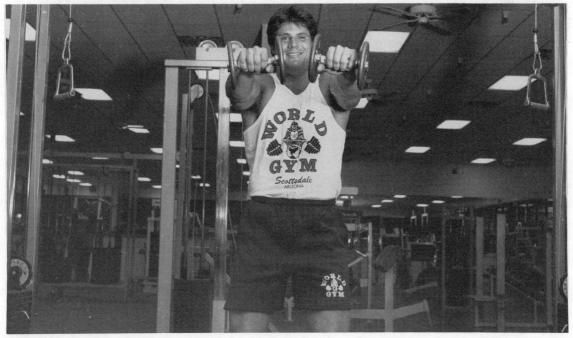

Posterior (Back) Dumbbell Raises (Double-Arms)

15 This is work for the rear or posterior deltoids in the shoulders. With slightly bent knees, bend over while arching the back. The back should be parallel to the floor, dumbbells hanging in front with the palms facing each other. With a slight bend in the elbows (which are facing the floor), raise the dumbbells out to a direct line at the height of the ears. Be careful here to notice if the dumbbells angle back. If so, then the deltoids will not get the work, because the back will take over.

15 START

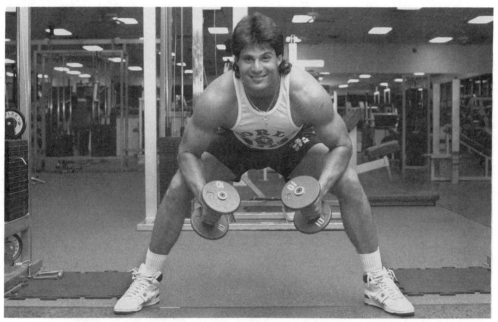

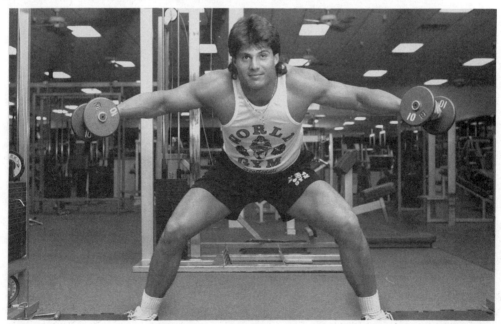

15 FINISH

Lateral (Side) Dumbbell Raises (Single-Arm)

16 These lifts work in the same general way as the posterior dumbbell raises described above, except that you use only one arm. The design of this lift is such that it should enable you to use a heavier weight with more of a concentrated lift.

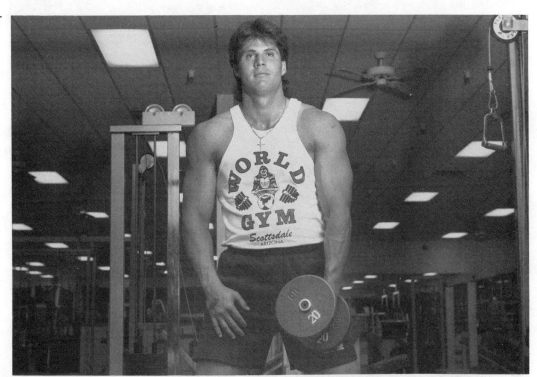

16 START

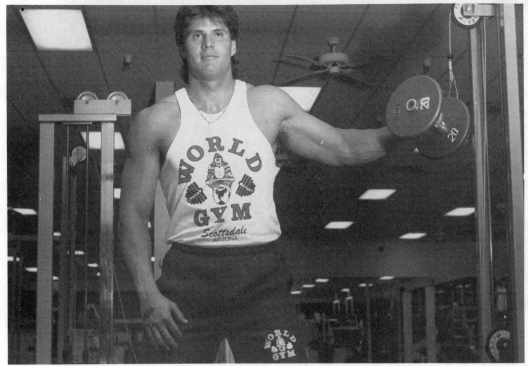

16 FINISH

Lateral (Side) Dumbbell Raises (Single-Arm)

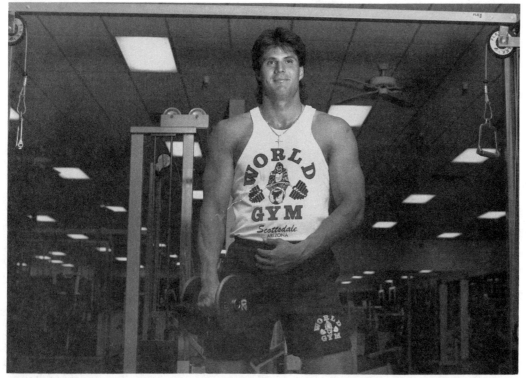

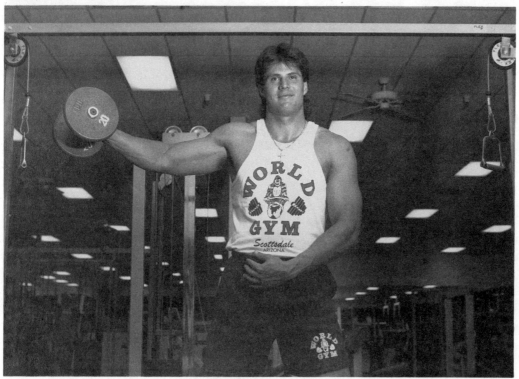

Anterior (Front) Dumbbell Raises (Single-Arm)

17 Instead of working the side (or lateral) deltoids as in (16), this routine works the front (or anterior) deltoids, as I am demonstrating.

17 START

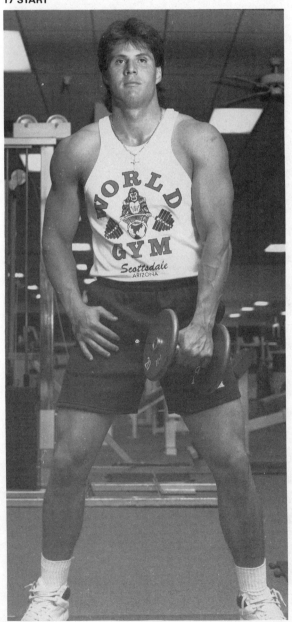

17 FINISH

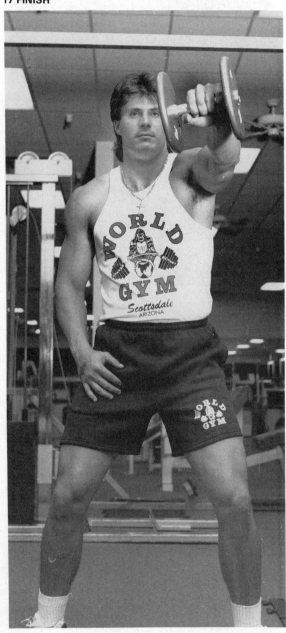

Anterior (Front) Dumbbell Raises (Single-Arm)

17 START

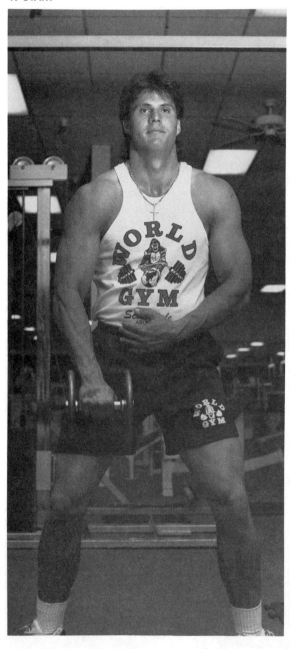

17 FINISH

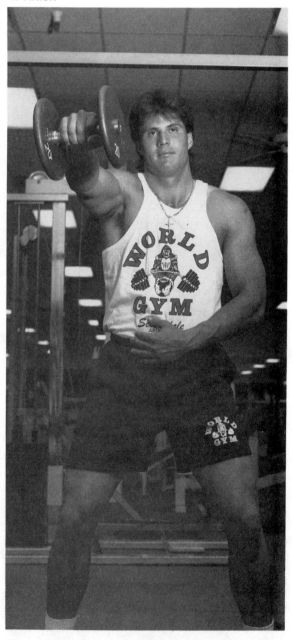

Posterior (Back) Dumbbell Raises (Single-Arm)

18 For the back deltoids, this routine is much like a dumbbell row, except that the grip on the dumbbells is with the palms facing back and the dumbbell is held away from the body. The elbows should be up and out while the forearm is straight up throughout the entire motion. Raise the dumbbell until the triceps are parallel to the floor. Pause and then lower the dumbbell, keeping it out away from the body.

18 FINISH

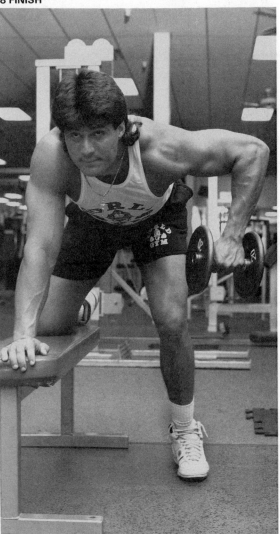

18 START

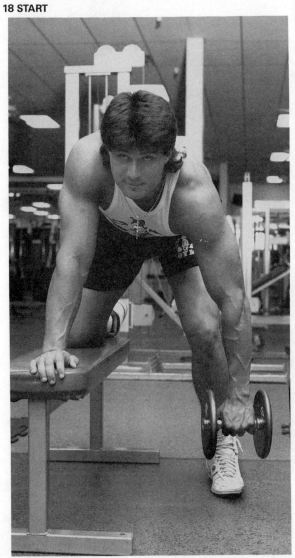

Posterior (Back) Dumbbell Raises (Single-Arm)

18 Good work for the back deltoids, this is much like a dumbbell row, only the grip on the dumbbell is palms facing back and the dumbbell is held away from the body with elbows up and out and forearm straight up throughout the entire motion. Raise the dumbbell until the triceps are parallel to the floor, pause, then lower dumbbell as I am doing, keeping it out away from the body.

At this point, I suggest that when you are using dumbbells you tip them for a little more deltoid (shoulder) involvement. For instance, refer back to (13) and (14) lateral and anterior. In any of these lifts, just presume that the dumbbell is filled with water and you are tipping them by rotating the shoulders at the peak of the lift so that the water would run out the front end of the dumbbell. Then lower in the normal manner.

18 START

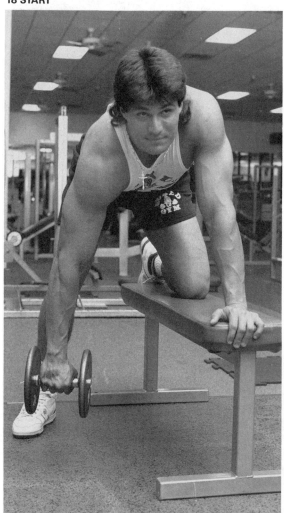

18 FINISH

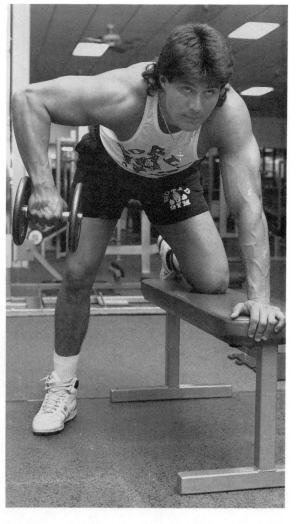

19 This routine works mainly the triceps. Lie on the bench with your head off the back of the bench as if you were looking back. With a close grip and holding the bar directly above your face, lower the bar to your forehead and push back up. Because the head is off the bench, the triceps will be forced to angle back, which will keep the tension on the triceps. If the triceps come upright to forward, the weight shifts off them. Thus, try to keep the angle of the triceps still. When pushing up, keep the elbows in. If you have trouble keeping your back flat on the bench, put your feet up on the bench. Breathe in coming to the forehead and blow out when pushing up.

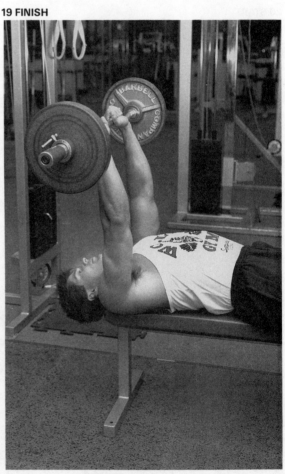

19 FINISH

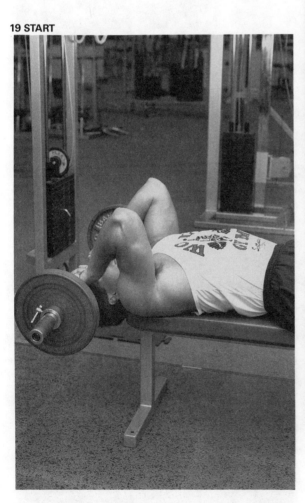

19 START

Tricep Press-Downs (V-Bar)

20 This routine also works mainly the triceps. Standing just back of the hanging grip, grab the grip with palms facing away. Keep your elbows at your side in the starting position, with the forearms parallel to the floor. In a semicircle away from the body, push the V-bar down to an arms-straight position. Avoid movement back in your elbows and avoid leaning on the top of the bar. Coming up higher than forearms parallel to the floor will put stress on the inner area of the elbow and the outer area of the wrist. If you are more comfortable with one foot in front of the other in this routine, that is no problem. Breathe in going up and breathe out as you go into the press down.

20 START

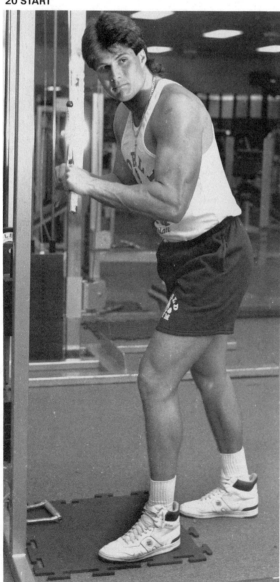

20 FINISH

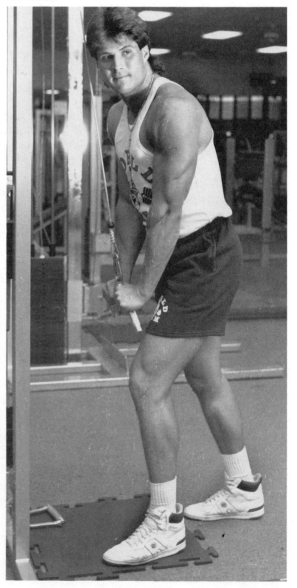

21 This is another tricep routine, except that it works mainly the outer tricep area. It is exactly the same as (20), except that when you pull the rope down, you flare out to the sides. Bring it in and back up to the forearms parallel to the floor position, as I show here.

21 FINISH

21 START

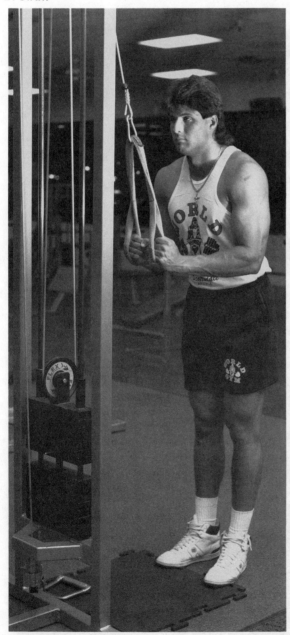

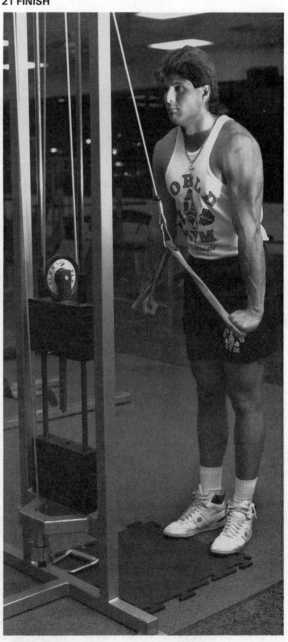

Tricep Bench Dips

22 Good work for the triceps. With palms less than shoulder width, grip the bench and elevate your feet about 6 inches higher than the hands. With back close to the bench, lower yourself to a point where you have a comfortable stretch in the shoulders and push up to an arms-fully-extended position. Do not lower too quickly; this can cause a strain in the shoulder. Lower slowly. Pause and then push back up. There is a tendency when doing work of this type to bounce on the bench. Do not bounce. Inhale as you lower and exhale on pushing up.

22 START

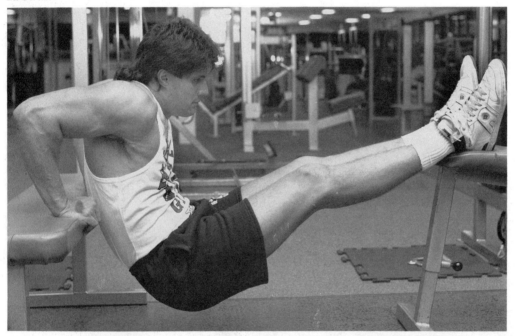

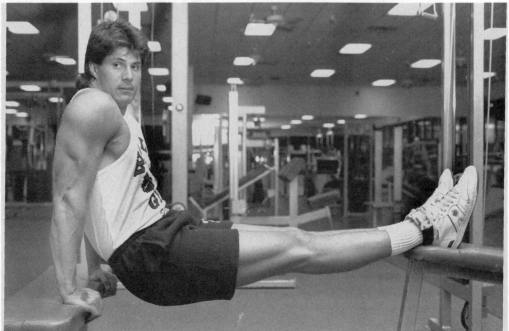

86

22 FINISH

23 With the back arched and straight, chin held up, lower until you feel a comfortable stretch in the shoulders, pause, and push back up. To help keep your balance, the legs should be bent and crossed. Leaning forward will transfer the weight from the triceps to the chest. Do this routine slowly and smoothly. Avoid bouncing, which (as noted above) can cause shoulder strain.

23 FINISH

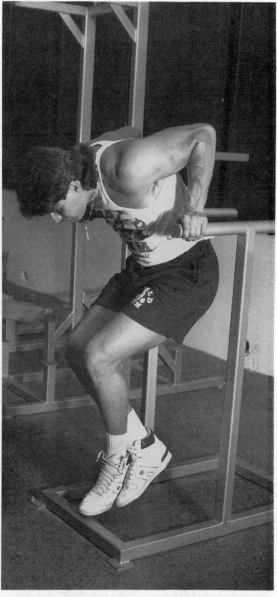

23 START

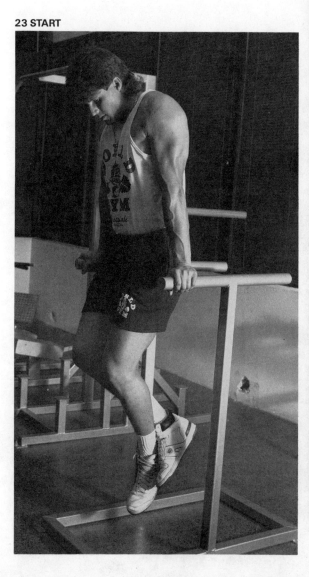

Tricep Kick-Backs

24 This routine concentrates on the inner tricep area and should only be performed at the end of your tricep workout. Bending over with the upper body parallel to the floor, put a hand on a bench to stabilize. Place a light dumbbell in your other hand, positioning your upper arm parallel to the floor alongside the upper body with the dumbbell hanging straight down toward the floor. With the dumbbell facing in, raise and twist (pronate) your arm so that the palms end facing upward. As you lower, twist (supinate) the dumbbell back to the starting position. It is important to concentrate on keeping the elbow still throughout this movement.

24 START

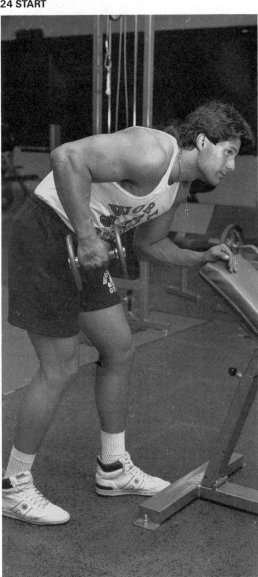

24 FINISH

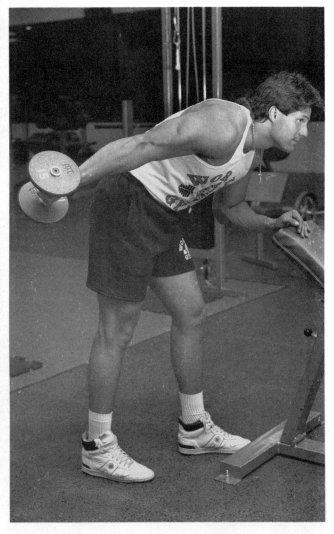

25 This routine works mainly with the triceps. Stand with your back to a shoulder level or overhead single-grip pulley. With the right arm in an L position, hold the grip with palms facing straight ahead. With the left arm supporting the right, push the weight out to full extension, then slowly bring it back. Do not take the forearm back farther than straight up, because to do so will cause stress on the inner elbow. Throughout the lift, keep the elbow still. Switch arms and repeat. Breathe out as you push and in as you bring the weight back.

25 START

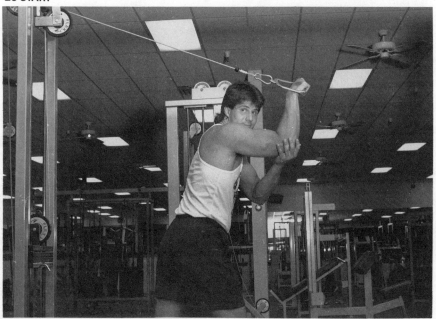

25 FINISH

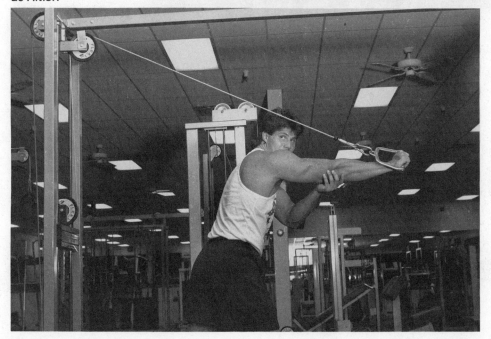

Overhead Tricep Extensions (Pulleys and V-Bar)

26 With your back to a shoulder-level or an above-the-shoulder-level pulley, grip the V-bar with your palms facing away. With the arms in an L shape, forearms straight up, push the weight out until the arms are fully extended. Bring the weight back to the ready position. Try not to bring the weight back too far past straight, because doing so places undue stress on the elbow. During the routine, keep tricep and elbow movement to an absolute minimum. Breathe out as you push out and in as you bring the weight back to the ready position.

26 START

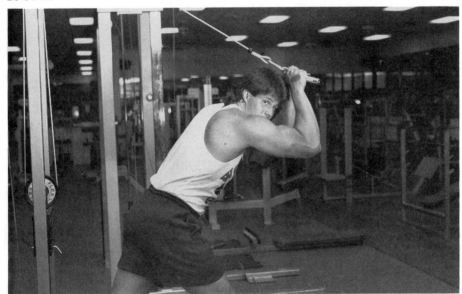

26 FINISH

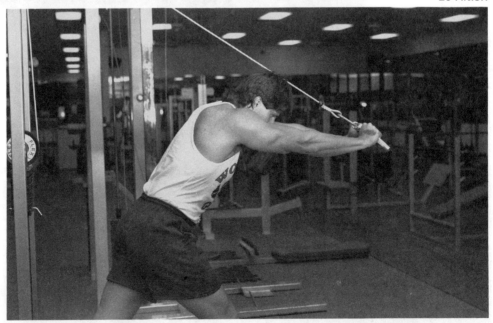

Closed-Grip Bench Press (Flat, Supine)

27 Still another tricep exercise. Start with the closer-than-shoulder-width grip on the bar. Keep your back flat on the bench, slowly lower the bar down to the sternum, and push straight up instead of angling back as in the regular bench press. Keep the elbows close to your sides and parallel to each other throughout the routine. Avoid bouncing the bar off the sternum and concentrate on your breathing. Inhale as you lower the weight and exhale in the lift. Putting your feet up on the bench will help in keeping your back flat against the bench for those who have a tendency to use too much leg and arching of the back during the lift.

27 START

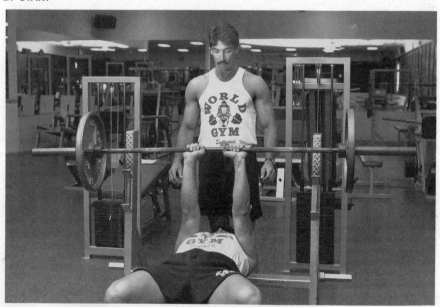

27 FINISH

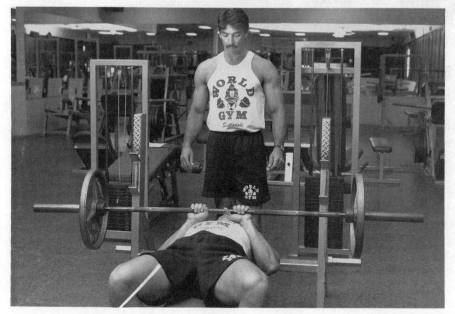

91

Scapular Rolls (Straight Lat Bar)

28 This works mainly the lats. This routine is done before any back exercise to exhaust the back without using the biceps. Use a straight lat bar with a shoulder-width grip facing away from you, as I am illustrating. With the shoulders and lats stretching as high as possible, pull down with the back bending at the elbows only slightly. You should feel nothing in the biceps. The lat bar should pull down only about 6 to 8 inches. Concentrate on the back doing the pulling. This movement should involve the shoulders coming down with shoulder blades coming together. There is a very slight lean backward in the lift.

28 START

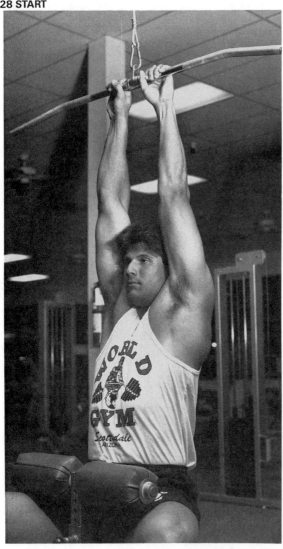

28 FINISH

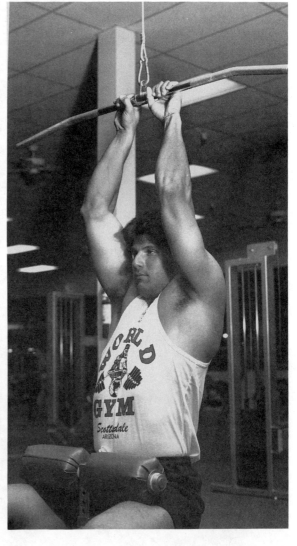

Wide-Grip Lat Pull-Downs (Behind Head)

29 Mainly for the upper lats, this routine begins with a wide grip on the lat bar, palms facing away from you. Position your body ahead of the bar to avoid hunching over when pulling the bar down behind the head to the base of the neck. Keeping the back straight, raise until you feel a stretch in the lats, and then pull down with concentration on the back.

29 FINISH

29 START

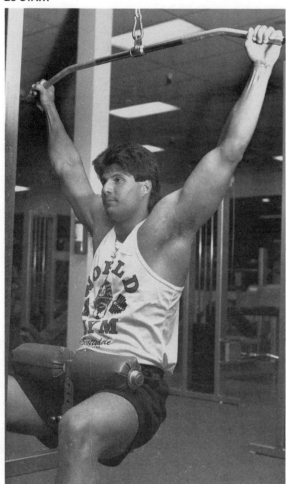

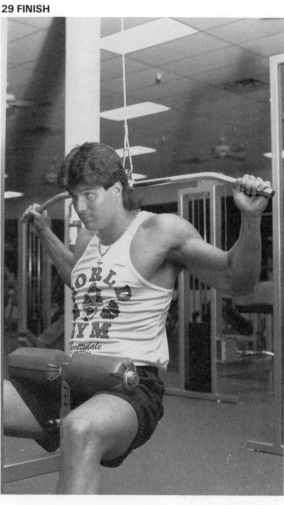

Wide-Grip Lat Pull Downs (To Chest)

30 Working mainly the middle lats, this routine also begins with a wide grip on the lat bar. Position your body under the lat bar, as I am showing, avoiding more than a slight leaning back when pulling the bar down to the chest. With arm extended, feeling a stretch in the back, pull down to an expanded chest. Feel the shoulder blades come together, raise, and repeat. Again, the palms are facing away in this routine.

30 START

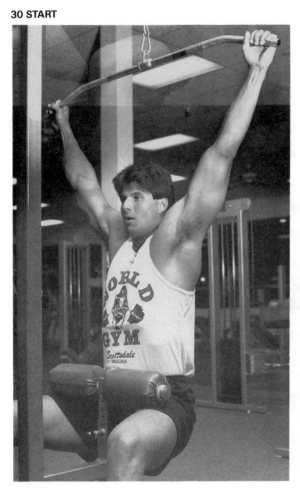

30 FINISH

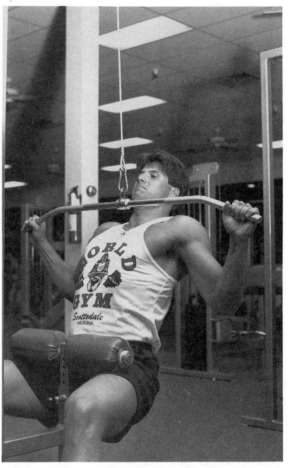

31 For working mainly the lower lats. Take a shoulder-width grip on the bar with palms facing toward you. With arms extended and feeling a stretch in the lats, pull the bar down to the sternum, keeping the elbows in and close to your sides. Expand the chest as you pull the weight down, pinching the shoulder blades together. As in (33), position yourself directly under the lat bar. Remember your breathing as in all routines.

31 FINISH

31 START

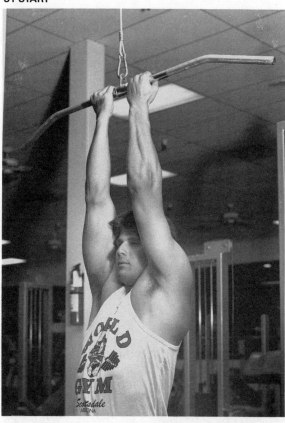

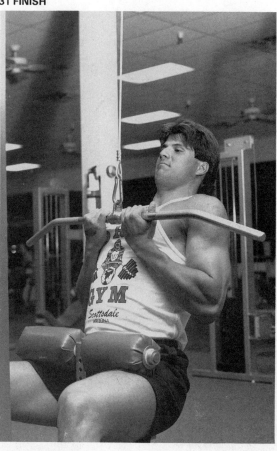

32 This routine works the whole lat (latissimus dorsi, teres major and minor, center and lower traps). Position yourself just behind the double grip. With a slight lean back, reach up and grab the grip. Feel the stretch in the back with arms extended. As you begin to pull the grip down, start leaning to about a 45-degree angle back at the same time. In one motion, you thrust the chest out to meet the grip. Keep the elbows close to the sides. In one motion, reverse the routine until the arms are extended back to a ready position. At ready position, feel the stretch, breathing out as you pull down and in as you bring the weight back up.

32 START

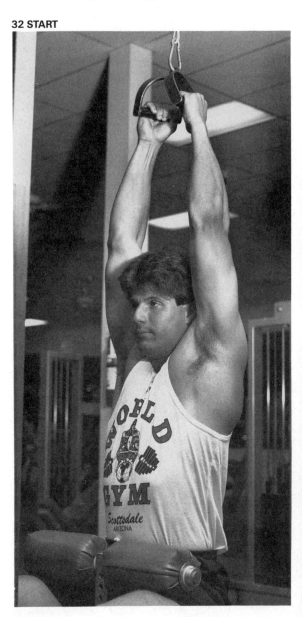

32 FINISH

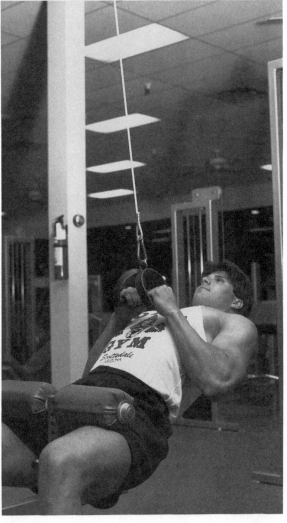

33 Working mainly the lower lats and center traps, this routine begins in a seated position. Once seated, your knees should be slightly bent. Then lean forward and grab the grip with the right hand. Palms should be facing down. Feel the stretch in the lat as you pull back. Rotate the grip until you have your palms facing your sides, elbows going no farther back than your sides (your bicep should end up straight up and down). As you pull back, your upper body comes up into a slightly leaning-back position. Think and feel the lat doing the work. The object here is to try to feel as though you're pulling the shoulder blade to the spine. Reverse hands and repeat.

33 START

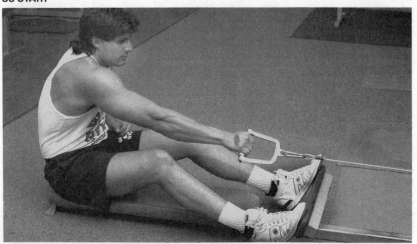

33 FINISH

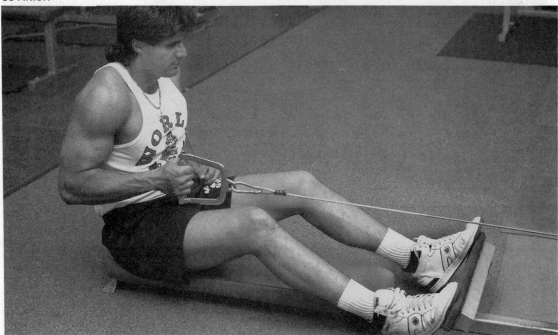

Single-Handed Low Lat Pulls (Pulleys)

33   The reason we use a single-hand grip instead of a double-hand grip here is that it allows you to deal with half the weight, putting far less strain on the lumbosacral joint of the lower back, and also provides a more concentrated effort on the lat.

33 START

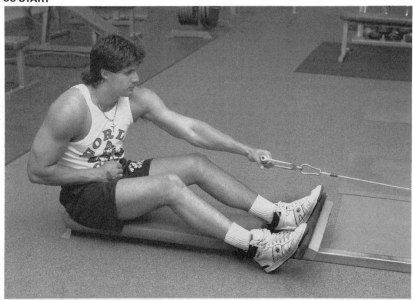

33 FINISH

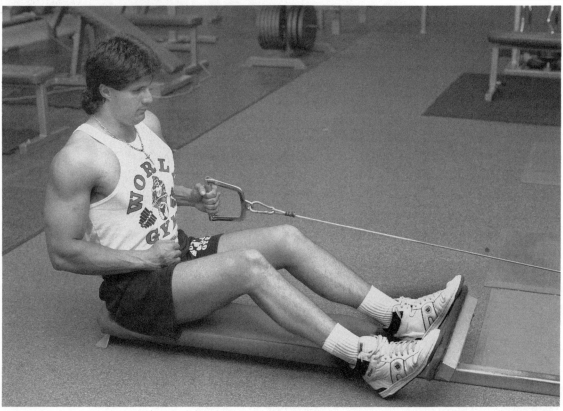

Bent-Over Rows (Dumbbells)

34 This routine works mainly the lats but also the center and lower traps, and teres major and minor. Bending over with one knee and hand supporting your body on a bench, arch the back. Hold the dumbbell slightly in front of you with palms facing back. All in one motion, as you pull the dumbbell up, rotate your hand to finish with palms facing your sides, elbows at your sides and no higher. Avoid flaring your arms out. Then lower and repeat. Breathe here as in all routines.

34 START

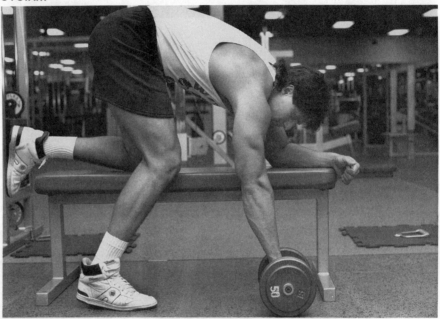

34 FINISH

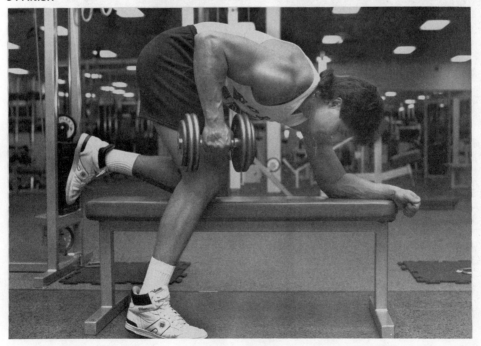

Bent-Over Rows (Dumbbells)

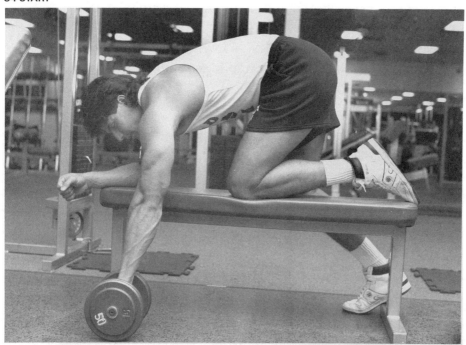

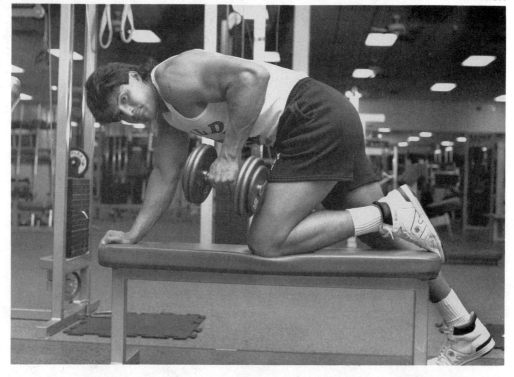

Hyperextensions (Roman Chair)

35 This work is mainly for the spinal erectors. With the upper body well out over the edge of the bench, elbows out and hands resting against the ears, hang with the body straight down as I am showing. Keep the chin up and the back arched, slowly raising the upper body until it is just above parallel to the floor. Slowly lower and repeat. Avoid using momentum to lift the body. Keep tensions in the spinal erectors throughout the lift. Do not push or overwork this area.

35 START

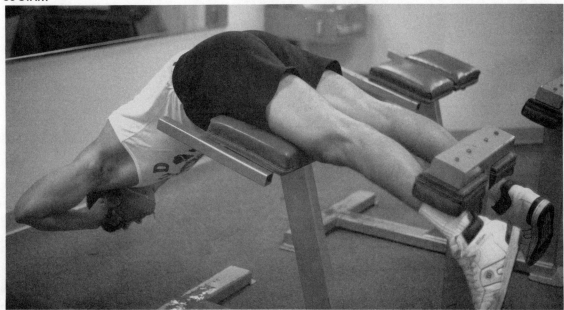

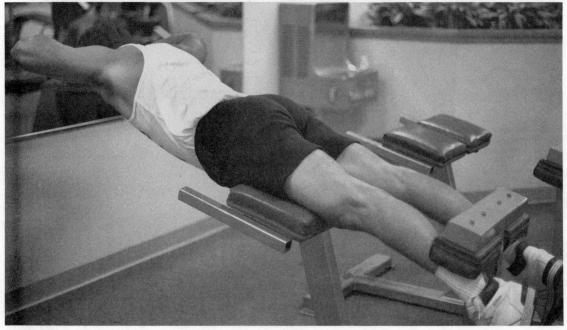

35 FINISH

Hyperextensions (Lying Down)

36 Again, work mainly for the spinal erectors. Lying on the floor with calves resting on a bench, place hands out to your sides and palms flat on the floor, raise the pelvis straight up as high as possible, and hold for a split second. Lower and repeat. Avoid using the arms to help in the lift. This routine is easier than the Roman chair version and is a good routine for those either not quite ready for the Roman chair or those with minor lower-back discomfort.

36A

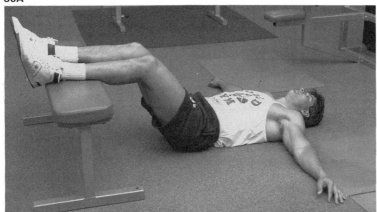

36B

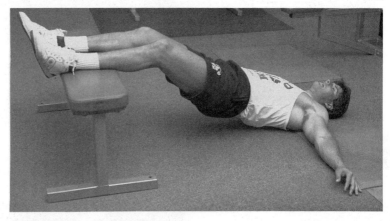

36C

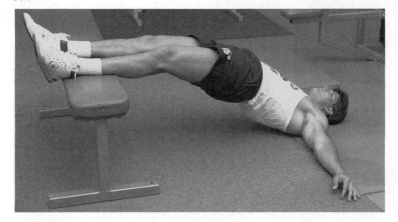

37 Works mainly the biceps. Hook a small EZ Curl bar up to a cable. Put the preacher-curl bench in front of the cables. The portion of your triceps just above the elbow should rest on the top part of the pad. Take a narrower-than-shoulder-width grip on the bar. You should have space between your underarms and the bench. With your head leaning slightly forward, curl the bar up to your chin. Keep your arms parallel to each other. Avoid leaning to help the weight up. Lower and repeat. Be sure that you have a narrower-than-shoulder-width grip, since it is important to keep the stress off the elbows. Concentrate on breathing throughout.

37 FINISH

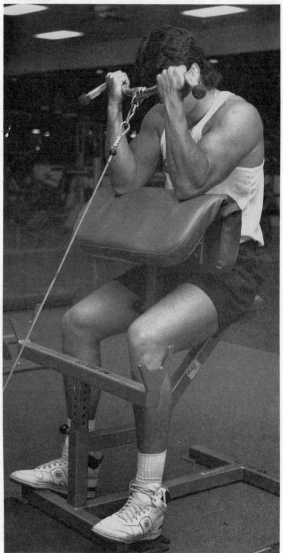

37 START

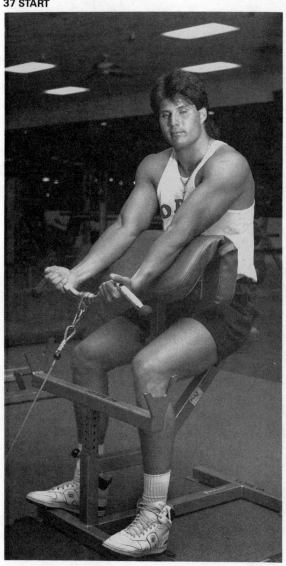

Preacher Curl (Preacher-Curl Bench)

38 This works mainly the biceps. Use an EZ Curl bar in the same manner as discussed in (37), except that when bringing the bar up, do not come all the way under the chin. Bring the bar up only as far as you are able to keep tension on the biceps. Coming up too high is a resting position with no tension on the biceps at all. You can't do as many reps, but you will get more out of the lift. Lower and repeat. Do not lean back. Elbows and forearms should be parallel to each other during the lift. Concentrate on breathing.

38 START

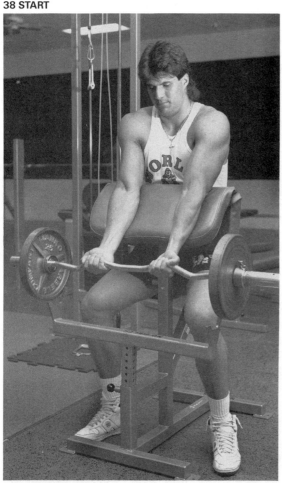

38 FINISH

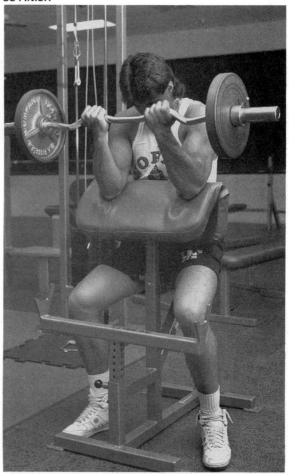

39 Works mainly the bicep. Standing with knees slightly bent and dumbbells at your side, palms facing back, with elbows a little forward, alternate hands while bringing the dumbbell up. Rotate your arm until, at the peak, the palms will be facing up. Rotate in the opposite direction as you lower the weight back to the starting position. Then repeat, using the other arm. Avoid letting the elbow go back during the lift. Try to raise and lower the weight in a straight line. To eliminate the potential for stress on the back, lean against a wall with the knees slightly bent.

39 FINISH

39 START

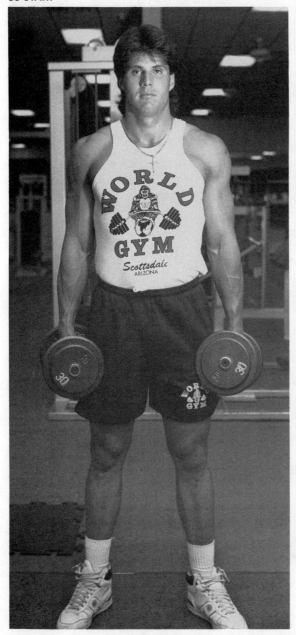
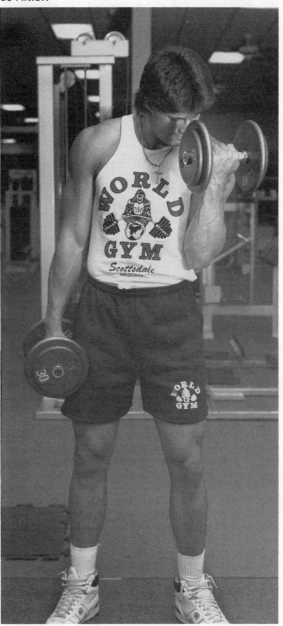

Standing Alternate Dumbbell Curls

39 START

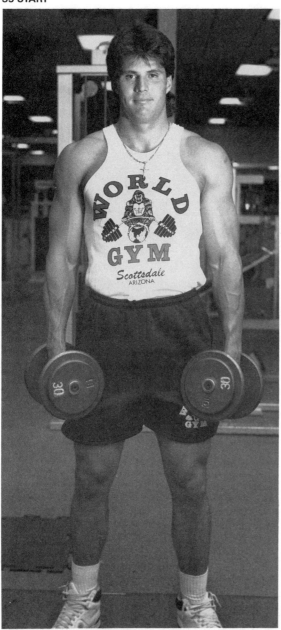

39 FINISH

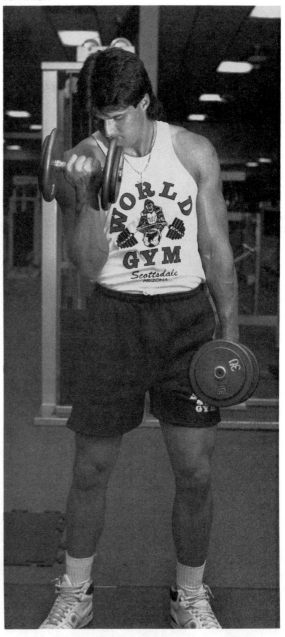

40 Works mainly the biceps. Sit at the end of a bench with your legs spread. Rest the right elbow just above the knee. As you bend over, palm facing the opposite leg, raise the dumbbell up to the right shoulder, rotating the forearms in. Lower and repeat. Do not let the elbow slip toward the groin area. If this happens, the lift will not be on a straight line and will put unwanted stress on the elbow. Do not lean back to help get the weight up.

40 FINISH

40 START

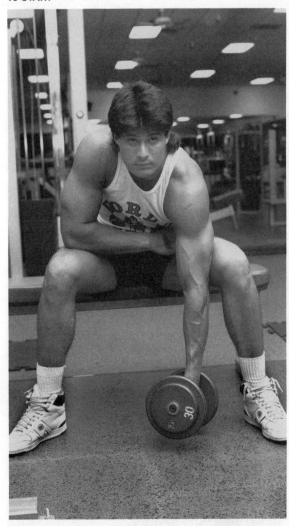

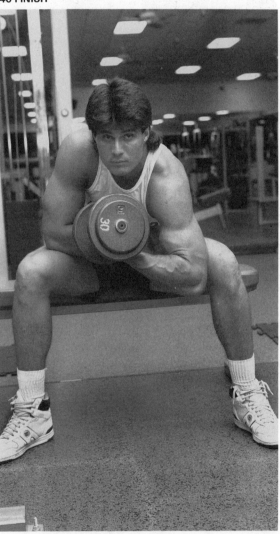

Concentration Curls

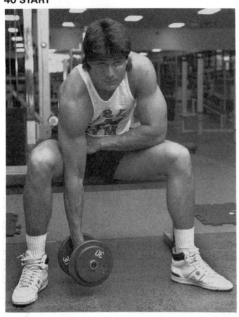

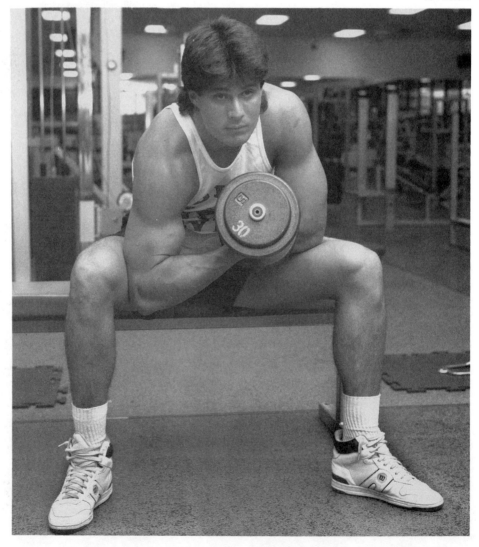

41 Works mainly the biceps. Seated on an incline bench with dumbbells hanging straight, have your palms facing in. Keep your legs close together (or crossed at the ankles) to enable you to raise the dumbbell straight up. Your first movement is arms straight and then bending at the elbows. Curl the dumbbell up, supinating during the lift until the palms finish facing forward on up. In the opposite direction, slowly lower the dumbbell back to the ready position. Now repeat with the other arm. Curl the weight up to the shoulder and back down.

41 START

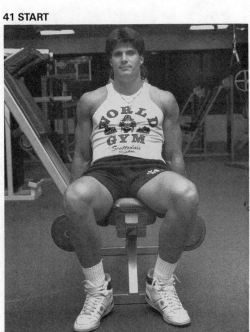

41 START

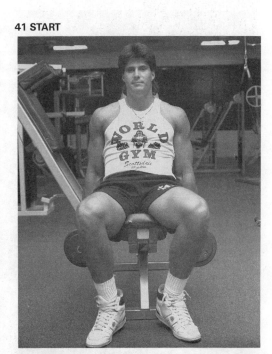

41 FINISH

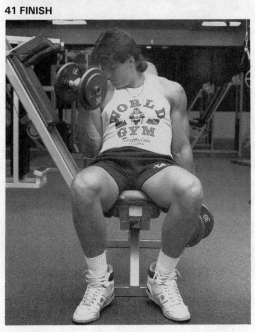

41 FINISH

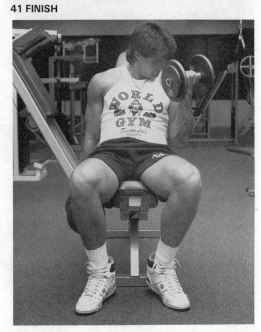

Standing Alternate Hammer Curls (Dumbbells)

42 Works mainly the biceps. Standing with legs either together or shoulder width apart, bend the knees slightly. Hold the dumbbells at your sides with palms facing in, as I am demonstrating. Alternating arms, raise one of the dumbbells, starting with arms straight and then bending at the elbows. Curl the weight up to the shoulder. Lower slowly and then repeat with the other arm. Keep from leaning back and avoid a rocking motion in the upper body.

42 START

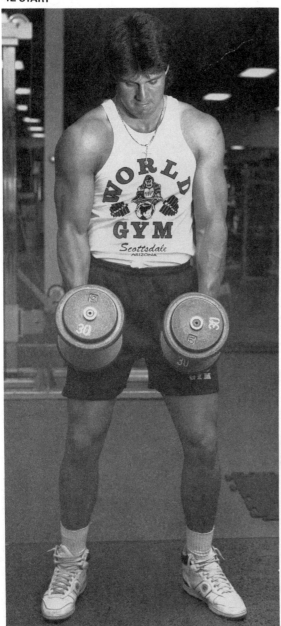

42 FINISH

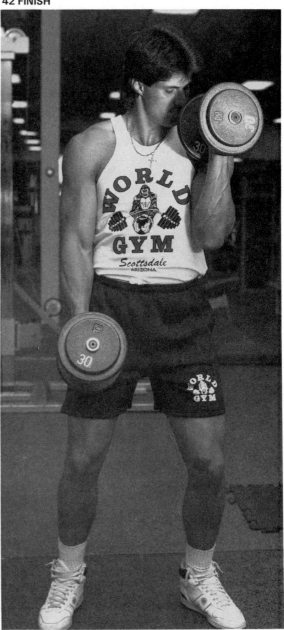

42 START

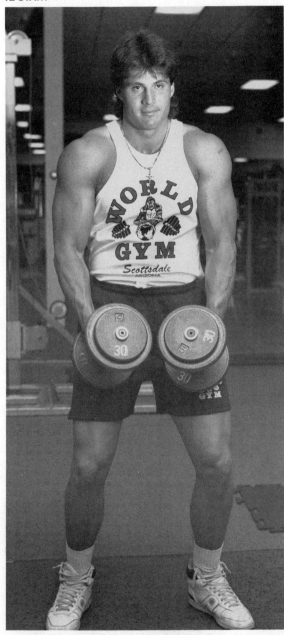

42 FINISH

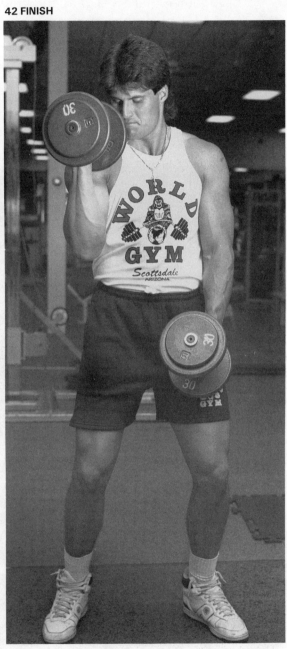

Standing Preacher Curls (EZ Curl Bar)

43 Works mainly the biceps. Standing with legs either shoulder width apart or together, make a slight bend in the knees. Take a less-than-shoulder-width grip on the bar. Keep the elbow as still as possible. Curl the weight up in front of the face. Lower slowly and repeat. Again, avoid any rocking motion or leaning back in the upper body. There is a natural tendency to do this. Concentrate on perfect form and technique. Placing your back against a wall will help support the back during lift. Do this if you wish. Concentrate on biceps and breathe. Your grip should have the palms facing in slightly.

43 START

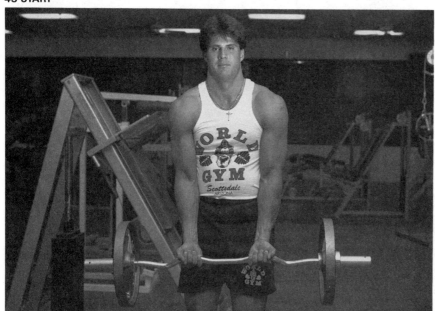

43 FINISH

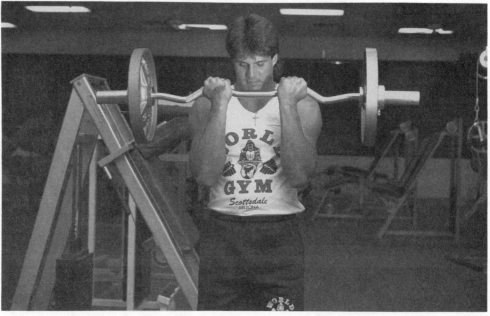

44 Works mainly the front and back part of the forearms (wrist flexors and extensors). With a shoulder-width grip on an Olympic bar, palms facing in, stand straight up. Relaxing the shoulders, arms fully extended, let the bar hang. With movement just in the wrist, rock the bar, rotating it toward you and out away from you. Do not hunch in the shoulders. Instead, relax the shoulders and let the bar hang. This is a very safe and quick way to work the forearms. Forearms, by the way, are among the more significant muscle groups for baseball.

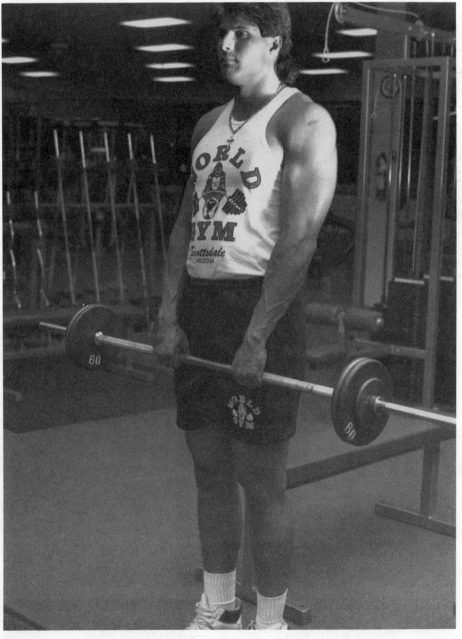

44 START

Standing Wrist Rolls

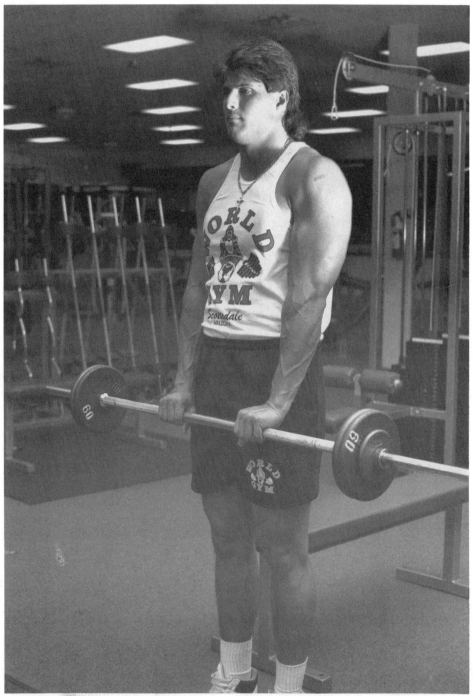

44 FINISH

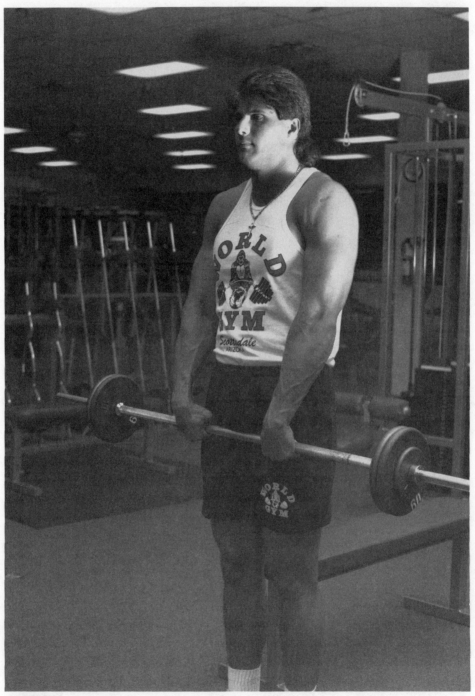

44 FINISH

Wrist Curls (Straight Bar)

45 Works mainly the inner forearm (wrist flexors). Straddling a bench, take a 6-inch grip on a bar with the palms facing away, as I am demonstrating. With the backs of the forearms resting on the edges of the bench, elbows staying about 6 inches apart just like the grip, move only in the wrist and curl the bar up to a palms-facing-up position. Lower slowly and repeat. Tip: Grip the bar tightly throughout this lift.

45 START

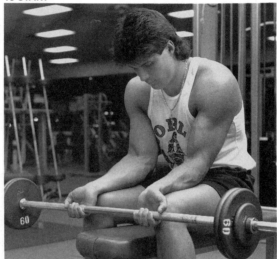

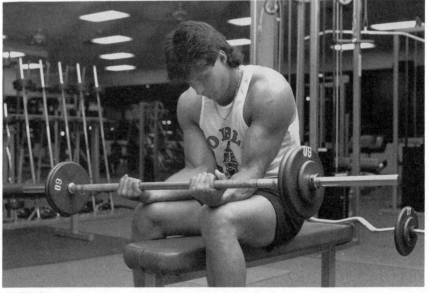

45 FINISH

46 Works mainly the back of the forearms. Again straddling a bench, take a shoulder-width grip on the bar with palms facing in. With the elbows resting on the legs just above the knees, get on your tiptoes to level out the position of the forearms. With movement only in the wrist, rotate the wrist upward until the palms are facing down. Lower and repeat. Lower the bar slowly and grip the bar tightly throughout the motion.

46 START

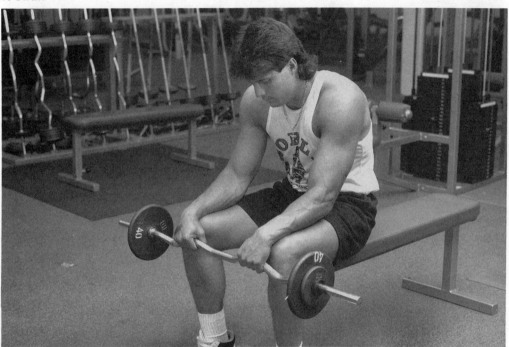

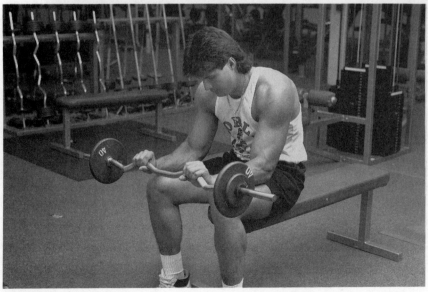

46 FINISH

Behind-The-Back Wrist Curls (Straight Bar)

47 Works mainly the inner part of the forearm. Place the bar across the end of a bench. Straddling the bench, bend over and pick up the bar with a shoulder-width grip, palms facing away from your body. As you bend forward, the inner forearms should rest against the top of the buttocks. Holding the bar tight, curl the bar up with movement of the wrist only. Lower slowly and repeat.

47 START

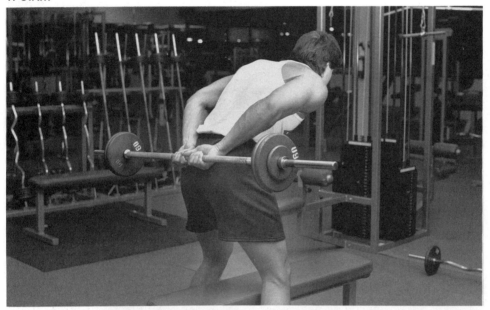

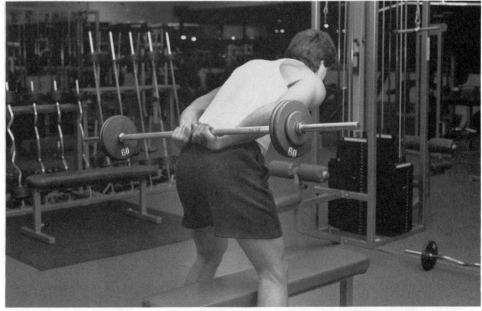

47 FINISH

48 Works mainly the back part of the forearms. Stand with knees slightly bent and a shoulder-width grip on the bar, palms facing in. Use movement only in the arms, curl the bar up to the chest, lower, and repeat. Avoid any rocking motion to help the weight up. Do not allow the elbows to flare out. Breathe.

48 FINISH

48 START

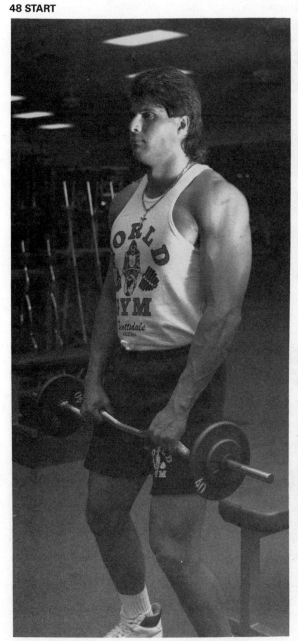
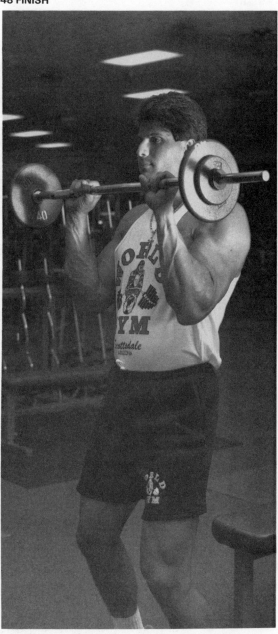

Wrist Abduction (Wrist Abductors)

49 Works mainly the outer forearms. Standing straight up, holding the unplated end of a dumbbell, extend your arms down. With movement in the wrist only, curl the weight up in a straight line as high as possible and then slowly lower to the ready position.

49 START

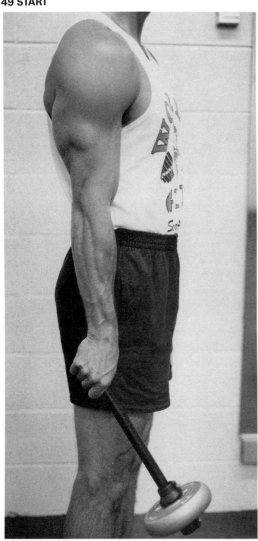

49 FINISH

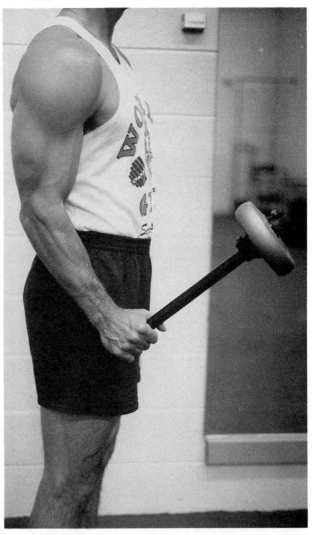

50 Works mainly the inner forearms. This is the same routine as (49), except that the weight is now behind you. With a tight grip, curl the weight up as high as possible and lower back to the ready position.

50 FINISH

50 START

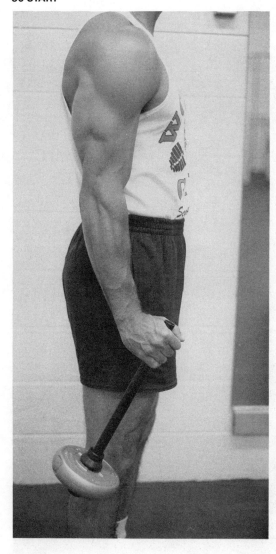

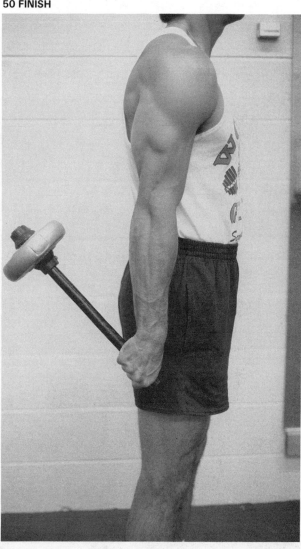

51 This is designed to work the finger flexor and extensor muscles in the forearms, the portions of the forearms needed for strong hands. This should always be the last upper-body routine of the day. Bend over, arching your back, and take a grip on the bar either straight on or similar to the grip on a baseball bat. Concentrate on using all the fingers and the thumb. Squeeze the fingers into a fist, raising the weight. Slowly lower and repeat.

51 START

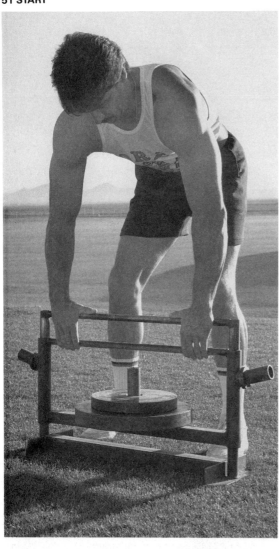

51 FINISH

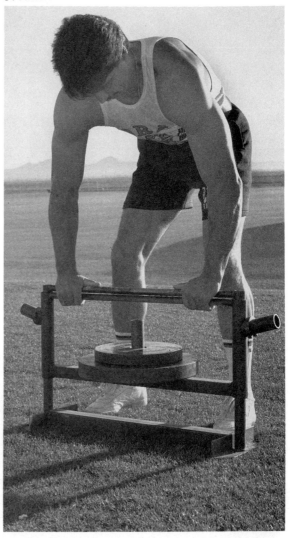

51 START

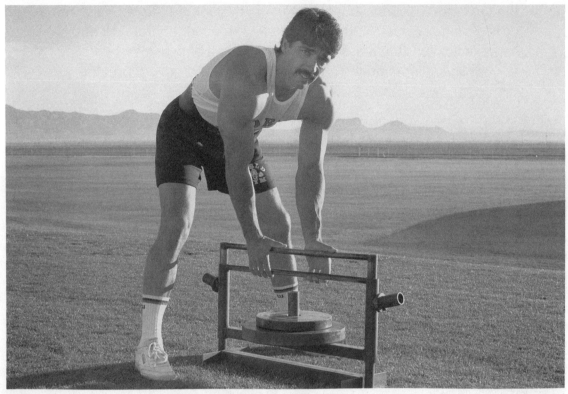

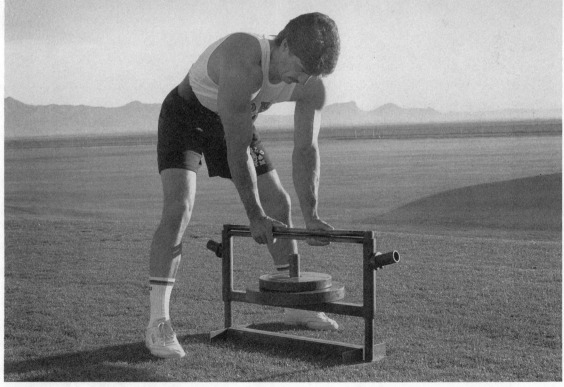

51 FINISH

Leg Extensions (Leg-Extension Machine)

52 Works mainly the outer quadriceps. Sitting on the machine, lean back with the toes pointed. Keep your toes pointed throughout the lift. Raise the weight until the legs are just short of being fully extended (do not lock out). At the same time, with little pressure, have the feeling of separating the legs. This will put added work on the outer quad. Lower and repeat. Breathe.

52 START

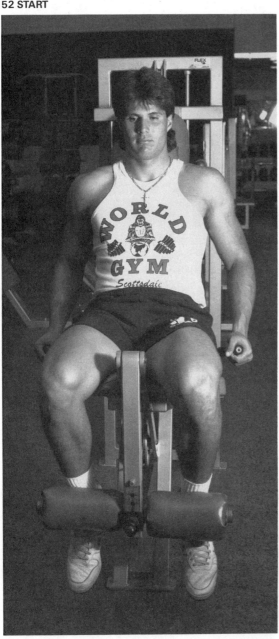

52 FINISH

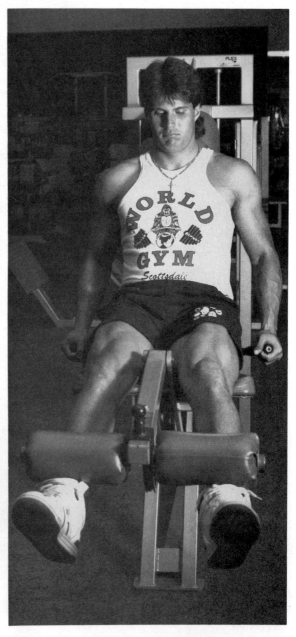

53 Works mainly the inner quadriceps. This routine is the same as (52), except that the upper body is leaning forward with the toes curled back. As you raise the weight, this time your concentration is on the quads coming together, which works the inner quads. Lower and repeat.

53 FINISH

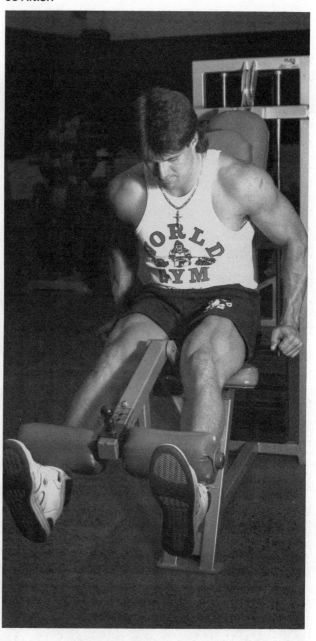

53 START

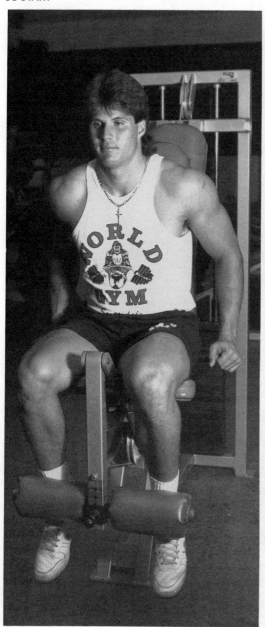

Leg Curls (Lying-Leg-Curl Machine)

54 Works mainly the leg bicep or hamstring. Here I'm lying down on a leg-curl machine with my pelvis pressing down against the bench. To do this routine, hold your head up and your chest flat against the bench. Hook your legs under the pads. Curl the weight as close to the buttocks as possible, keeping the hips down. The hamstring curl is effective only through proper form and technique. What is important here is the tension in the hamstring, not the amount of weight.

54 START

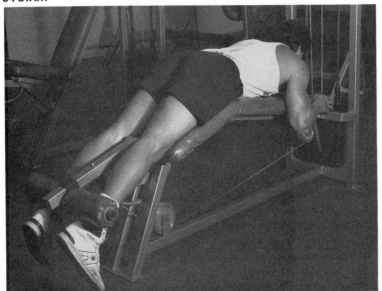

54 FINISH

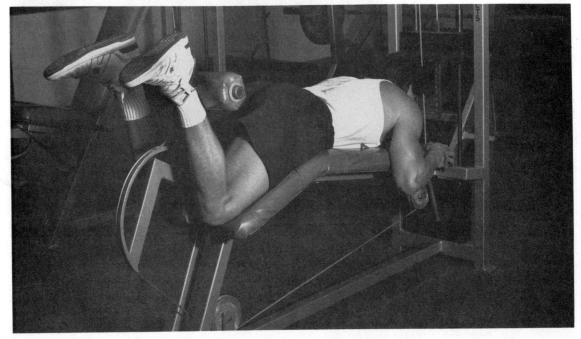

55 Another routine for the hamstring. More of a concentrated lift because of its single action, this routine is done standing. Rest the quads against the pads (one leg at a time), with the pad resting against the lower calf area. Curl the weight up with the heel as close to the buttocks as possible. During the lift, avoid any rocking motion in the upper body to help the weight up. This is better known as ''cheating.'' Our frequent references to these habits throughout this program are important. Cheating on a lift deprives you of the value of the lift. Always remember that perfect form and technique are the only way to go. Lift less weight if you have to. Do fewer reps if you have to. But don't ever cheat on a lift.

55 FINISH

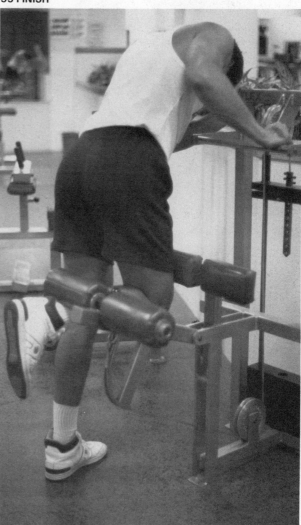

55 START

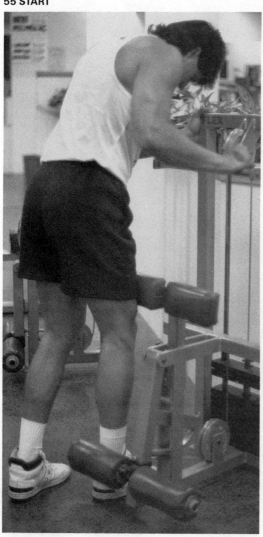

Standing Leg Curls (Standing-Leg-Curl Machine)

55 START

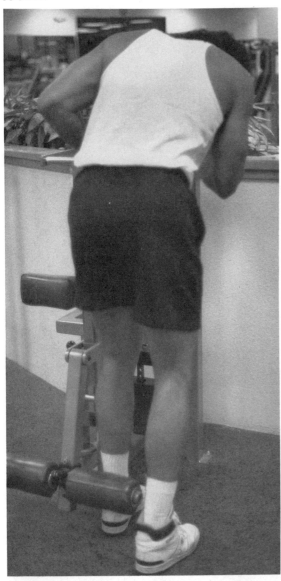

55 FINISH

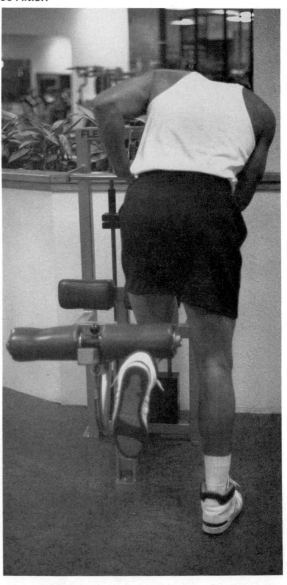

56 A great full-lower-body workout, concentrating mainly on the quads but also working the glutes and hamstrings. Seated comfortably with the feet at shoulder width, lower the weight down to about three-quarters squat or just a little more. Lowering into a full squat puts too much stress on the knees. Push the weight back up until the legs are just short of being fully extended (or locking out). Lower slowly and push up. Keep the upper body still throughout the motion. Breathe.

56 START

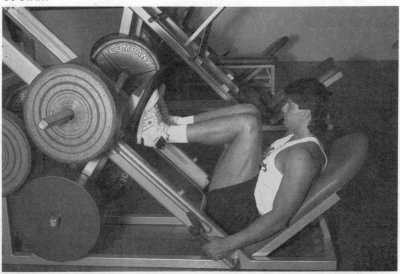

56 FINISH

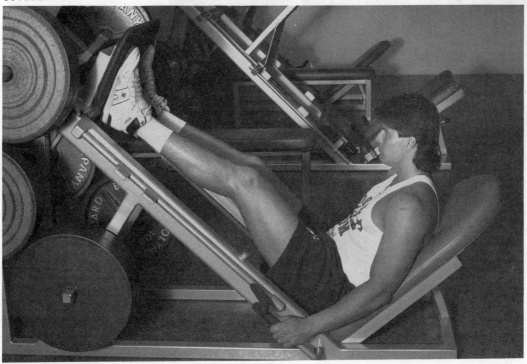

Lunges (Straight Bar)

57 This is another great full-lower-body workout, concentrating mainly on the hamstrings and buttocks but also on the quads and calves. Stand straight up with the weight on the upper back and shoulders. Alternating legs, step forward as far as comfortably possible with the right leg. The lower half of the leg should be straight up. Too short a stride will put too much stress on the knees. The left knee should end up an inch or so from the floor. The back should be arched to keep the upper body straight up and not leaning forward during the lift. Push up into the starting position. Alternate legs, so that with the left leg doing the stride, the right knee will be about an inch or so from the floor.

57 START

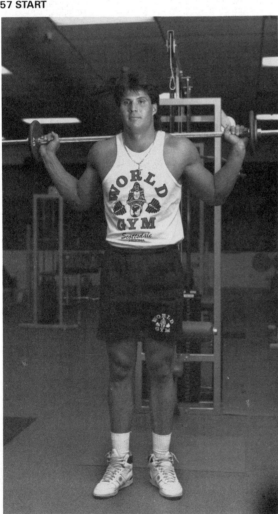

57 FINISH

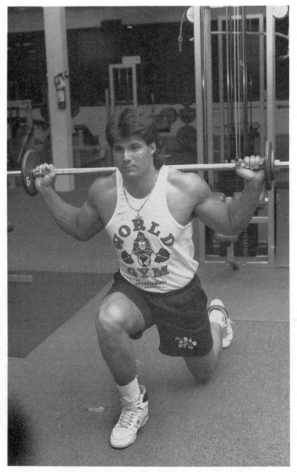

Lunges (Straight Bar)

57 FINISH

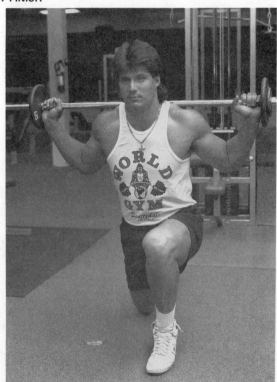

57 START

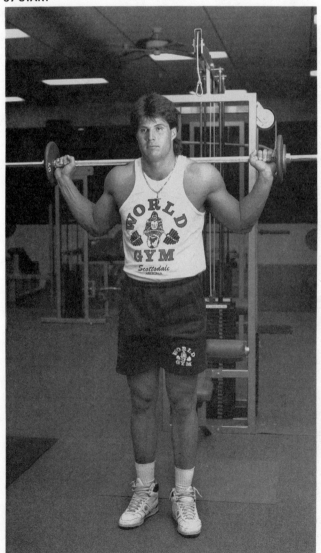

Calves (Hip Sled or Universal)

58 This sequence works the medial (inside), lateral (outside), and middle calf. **58A** Seated with back supported, put the balls of both feet on the bottom of the foot plate (feet should be straight up). Push the legs out (and weight up) until both legs are fully extended. Start the routine by pushing the toes forward and bringing them all the way back. This is a routine that you should work into gradually. Avoid the tendency to overwork in the first two or three workouts.

58 A

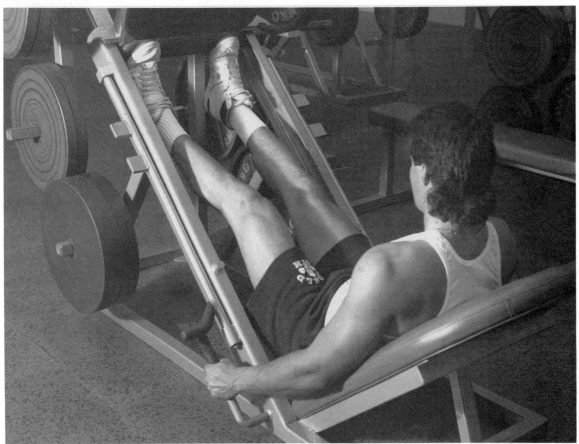

58B This is done the same way as the straight routine, except that the feet are angled with toes together and heels apart.

58 B

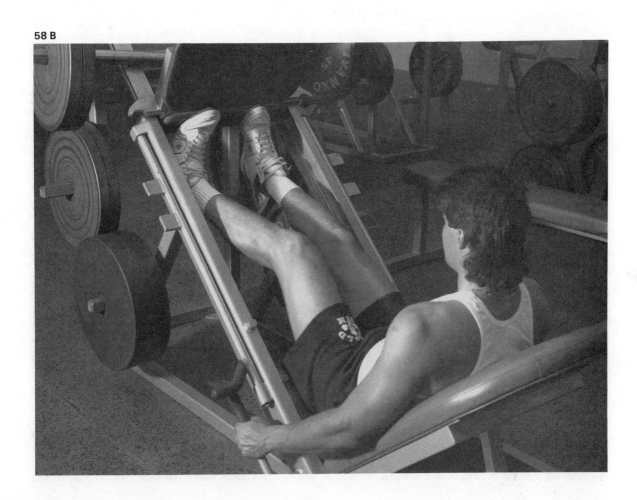

Calves Out

58C Now the routine is done the same way, except that the heels are together and the toes are angled outward.

58C

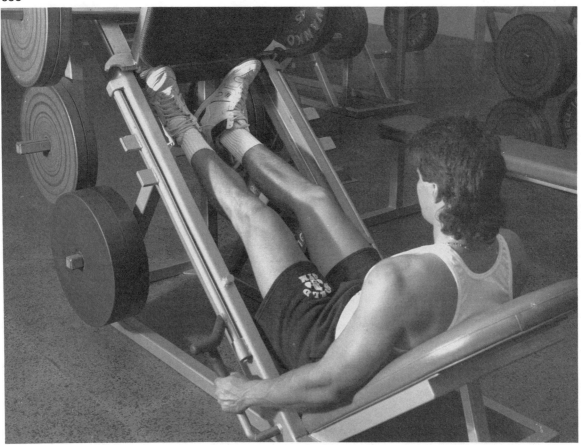

59 Again, we work through the three calf areas. Sit in the calf machine with the pad just above your knees, the balls of the feet on the step (but the heels not on the step). With the feet straight, lower your heels to where you feel the stretch, then push up onto your toes. Again, I caution you about overworking in the early going.

59A Feet are straight. This works the middle calf.

59A

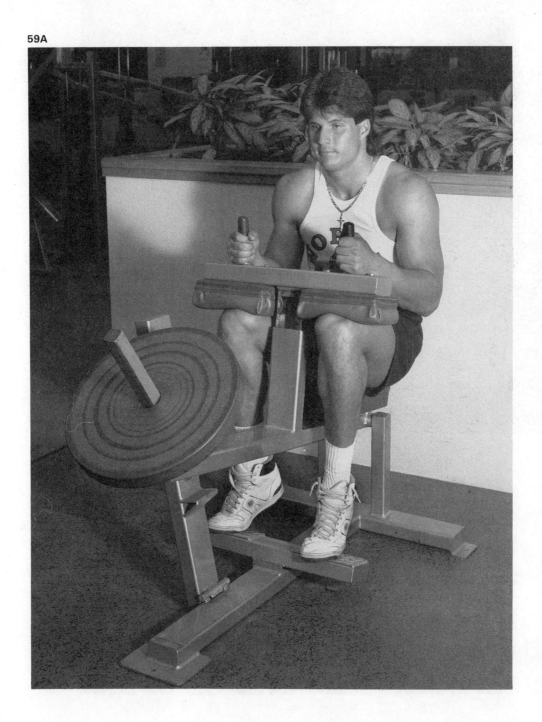

Seated Calf Machine (In)

59B To work the inner calf, do the same routine with the feet angled in (that is, toes together and heels apart).

59B

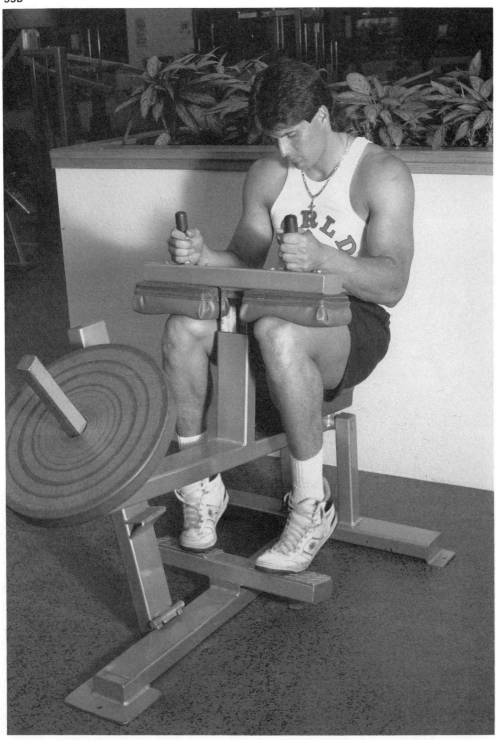

59C For the outer calf, the same routine, only this time the heels are together and the toes are angled out.

59C

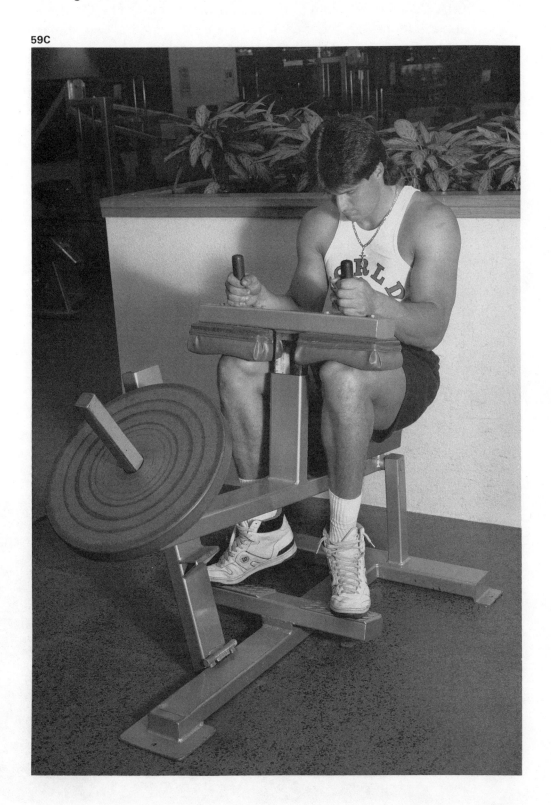

Donkey Calf Raises (Straight)

60 As with other calf routines, here we have a three-part position sequence for the middle, medial, and lateral calf.

60A Bending over with the pads and weight resting on the lower back (or the upper buttocks), place the balls of the feet on the bar with the heels off. Keeping the feet pointed straight ahead, lower the heels until you feel the stretch in the calves. Then raise up on your toes, lower, and repeat.

The advantages to the bent-over, rather than the upright, weight on the shoulders is that it allows you to eliminate the stress of the heavy weight on the upper back, which compresses the vertebrae.

60A START

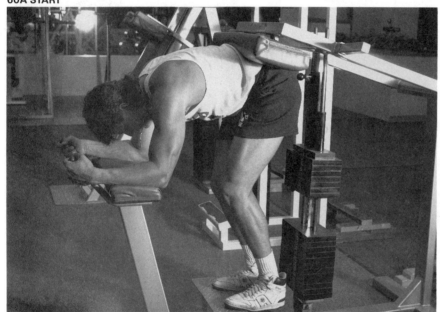

60A FINISH

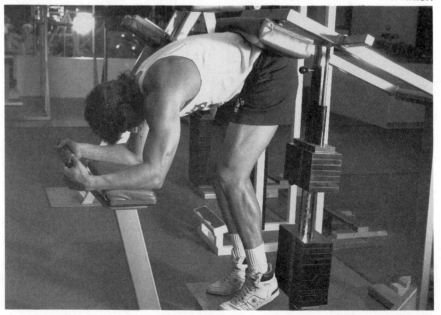

60B This is the same as the straight, but the feet are angled with the toes together and the heels apart.

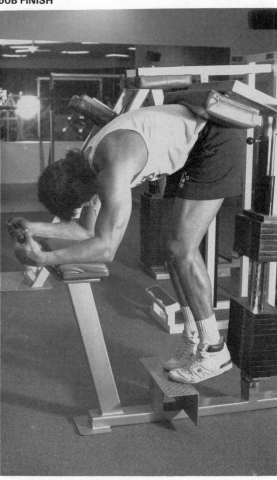

60B FINISH

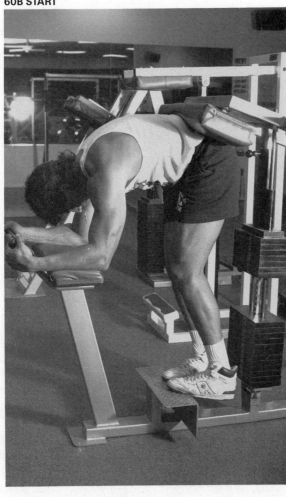

60B START

Donkey Calf Raises (Out)

60C The lateral calf work is done the same as the other forms, except that the feet are angled with the heels together and the toes pointed outward.

60C START

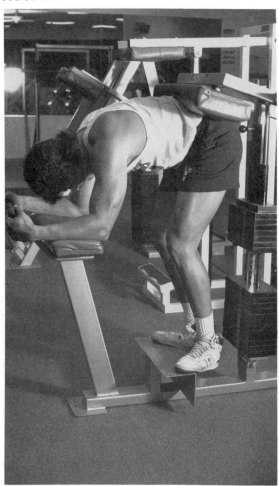

60C FINISH

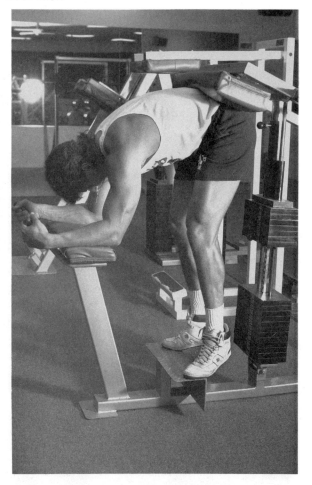

61 This exercise works the entire abdominal area. Sit in a Roman chair or on a bench with your feet under a bar. Fold your arms as I am doing and hold them out away from your chest. Concentrate on the abdominals only. Lower backward, tucking your chin into your chest. Lower down until the upper body is parallel with the floor. The movement must be slow, keeping the tension on the abs throughout the movement. Inhale and hold your breath as you lower your body. This not only puts added pressure on the abdominal muscles, but it also keeps the spine firm. Continue to hold your breath as you raise your back up. Then breathe. Holding your breath is useful any time you have to keep your spine erect.

61 START

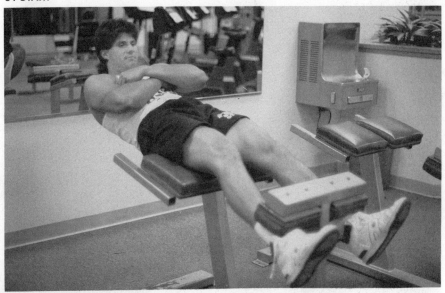

61 FINISH

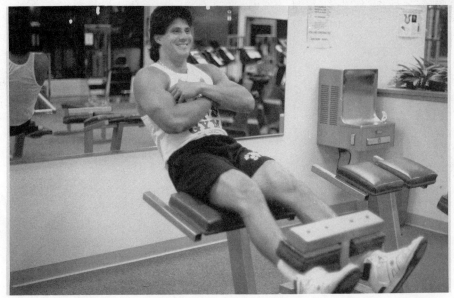

Twisters

62 Works mainly the spine and torso. To loosen up the lower to upper back. Start in a standing position with a slightly better than shoulder-width spread of the legs. Make a slight bend in the knees. Your arms should be held in an L shape. Rotate the body easily to first one side and then to the other side. Blow out at the completion of the twist. Start off easy, and as you continue your trunk will loosen up to the point where you can twist farther and farther. A comfortable and useful exercise for not only after your lift but also before.

62 START

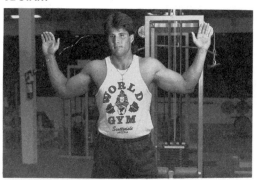

62 FINISH

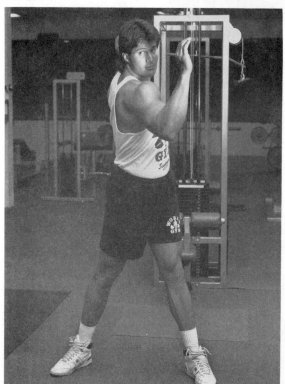

62 FINISH

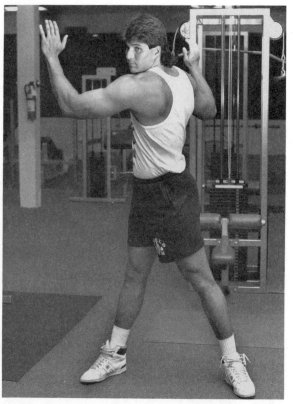

Now that you have seen all of the various routines that make up the program, it is important that you decide how to use it.

What we have done here is show you how the program is used by our team. Usage varies a bit from spring training to the regular season. One of the important elements to keep in mind is that there are times when the best thing you can do is take a day off. We have designed the program so that it contains easy days (or at least relatively easy).

But if you do not feel up to handling the program, especially if you have just completed a full cycle of the program you have selected, take a day to rest.

Do not lift at all if you are in pain. Even if you are experiencing mild discomfort, stop your program and go for a checkup. A muscle has only a hundred percent to give; it cannot give more than that. If a muscle is in pain, it is signaling to you that it is damaged. Don't damage it further. Muscles do break down in the natural course of developing. But they should do so without pain.

Basically, we have five programs to select from. We name them and design them for the baseball season, starting with off-season. They are:

1. Off-season program (3 days — primary)
2. Off-season program (3 days — alternate)
3. Off-season program (4 days) and (6 days)
4. Spring-training program (3 days)
5. In-season program (2 days)

You will see the term *supersetting* used in the programs. Supersetting is when you go from one lift to the other without any rest in between. You can sometimes superset the same muscle group or two different groups. The problem with supersetting is that in a busy gym, you will have trouble using two pieces of equipment at one time. If this is not possible, then do the two exercises separately.

Example:

SUPERSETS		SETS	REPS
Bench Press	together	3	8–10
Lat Pull-Downs	3 times		8–10

No SUPERSETS	SETS	REPS
Bench Press	3	8–10
Lat Pull-Downs	3	8–10

Supersetting makes for a quicker program.

Three-day Off-season Program

Day One: Monday
Day Two: Wednesday
Day Three: Friday

Day Two or Wednesday will be the easiest day.

Day One (Monday) and Day Three (Friday)

Stretch	Sets	Reps	Lbs.
1 Push-ups (Warm-up)	1		
3 Bench Press Supine	4	8–10	
7 Supine D.B. Flys	3	8–10	
6B Bench Press (Incline D.B.'s)	2	8–10	
*9 Cross-body Cable Pulls	3	8–10	
10 Military Press ⎤ Super Set	3	8–10	
12 Upright Rows ⎦		8–10	
43 Standing Preacher Curls	4	8–10	
39 Standing Alternate (Supinated) D.B. Curls	4	8–10	
41 Seated D.B. Curls (Incline)	4	8–10	
19 Lying French Press ⎤ One or the Other	3	8–10	
27 Closed-grip Bench Press ⎦	3	8–10	
20–21 Tricep Press-downs (Rope or V-bar) ⎤ Super Set	3	8–10	
22 Tricep Bench Dips ⎦		As many	
28 Scapular Rolls	1	As many	
29 Wide-grip Lat Pull-downs (Behind neck)	3	8–10	
30 Wide-grip Lat Pull-downs (To chest)	3	8–10	
31 Reverse Close-grip (To sternum)	3	8–10	
*33 Single-handed Low Lat Pulls ⎤ One or the Other	3	8–10	
*34 Bent-over Rows D.B.'s ⎦	3	8–10	
44 Standing Wrist Rolls	1 each way	40, 30, 25	
51 Gripper	2	As many	
52 Leg Extensions (Toes pointed)	3	13–15	
53 Leg Extensions (Toes back)	3	13–15	
54 Leg Curls	4	13–15	
56 ¾ Leg Press	4	13–15	
59A Seated Calf Machine (Straight)	2	20	
59B Seated Calf Machine (In)	2	20	
59C Seated Calf Machine (Out)	2	20	

Abs. 6″ Leg Raises	6″ Leg Raises	AB Crunches	¼ Sit-ups	side leg raises
15			30	
25 Reps (M)	20 Reps (M)	25 Reps (S)	As many (F)	10 Reps
Sec.			Sec.	

	Sets	Reps
62 Twisters	1	50

Stretch

* Optional

First Program

Day Two (Wednesday)

Stretch		Sets	Reps	Lbs.
1 Push-ups (Warm up)		1		
3 Bench Press Supine	} Super Set	3	10–12	
32 Close Grip Lat Pull-Downs			10–12	
36 Hyperextensions (Lying)	} One or the Other	2	20	
35 Hyperextensions (Roman chair)		2	12–15	
11 Seated Alternate D.B. Press	} Super Set	3	10–12	
12 Upright Rows			10–12	
37–38 Preacher Curls (Preacher Bar or Cables)	} Super Set	3	10–12	
20 Tricep Press-downs (V-bar)			10–12	
* 24 Tricep Kick-backs	} One or the Other	2	13–15	
* 23 Tricep Dips (Dip Bar)		2	As many	
44 Standing Wrist Rolls		1 each way	40, 30, 25	
51 Gripper		2	As many	
52 Leg Extensions (Toes Pointed)	} Super Set	3	13–15	
54 Leg Curls			13–15	
53 Leg Extensions (Toes Back)	} Super Set	2	13–15	
54 Leg Curls			13–15	
60A Calves (Straight)	*Donkey Calf Machine or Universal* 58A	2	20	
60B Calves (In)	*Donkey Calf Machine or Universal* 58B	2	20	
60C Calves (Out)	*Donkey Calf Machine or Universal* 58C	2	20	
61 Bench Sit-ups		2	As many	
62 Twisters		1	50	

Stretch

* Optional

3-Day Off-Season Program

Day One (Monday)   Day Three (Friday)

Stretch	Sets	Reps	Lbs.
1 Push-ups (Warm-up)	1		
3 Bench Press Supine	4	8–10	
7 Supine D.B. Flys	3	8–10	
8 Incline D.B. Flys	2	8–10	
9 Cross Body Cable Pulls *Option	3	8–10	
29 Wide Grip Lat Pull-Downs (Behind Head)	3	8–10	
30 Wide Grip Lat Pull-Downs (To Chest)	3	8–10	
31 Reverse Close Grip Pull-Downs (To Sternum)	3	8–10	
32 Close Grip Lat Pull-Downs	4	8–10	
33 Single Handed Low Lat Pull	3	8–10	
34 Bent Over Rows D.B.'s	3	8–10	
10 Military Press	3	8–10	
12 Upright Rows		8–10	
43 Standing Preacher Curls	4	8–10	
41 Seated Incline D.B. Curls	3	8–10	
40 Concentration Curls DB's	3	8–10	
19 Lying French Press	4	8–10	
27 Closed Grip Bench Press	4	8–10	
20 Tricep Press-downs (V bar or rope)	3	8–10	
22 Tricep Bench Dips		8–10	
44 Standing Wrist Rolls	1 each way	40, 30, 25	
51 Gripper	2	As many	
56 ¾ Leg Press	4	12–15	
52 Leg Extensions (Toes Pointed)	2	12–15	
53 Leg Extensions (Toes Back)	2	12–15	
54 Leg Curls	3	12–15	
59A Seated Calf Machine (Straight)	2	20	
59B Seated Calf Machine (In)	2	20	
59C Seated Calf Machine (Out)	2	20	

Monday: 29, 30, 31, 32 }

Not Both on same day } Friday: 33, 34

10 Military Press / 12 Upright Rows } Super Set

19 Lying French Press / 27 Closed Grip Bench Press } Not both on same day

20 Tricep Press-downs / 22 Tricep Bench Dips } Super Set

Abs. 6" Leg Raises	15	6" Leg Raises	AB Crunches	¼ Sit-ups	30	Side Leg Raises
25 Reps (M)	Sec.	20 Reps (M)	25 Reps (S)	As many (F)	Sec.	10 Reps

62 Twisters	1	50 each way

Stretch

Second Program

3 Day Off-Season Program

Day Two (Wednesday)

Stretch		Sets	Reps	Lbs.
1 Push-ups (Warm-up)		1		
6A Bench Press DB's Supine	} Super Set	3	8–10	
32 Close Grip Lat Pull-Downs			8–10	
39-38 Hyperextensions (36) Lying or (35) Roman Chair)		2	12–15	
16 Lateral Side D.B. Raises (Single arm)		2	8–10	
17 Anterior D.B. Raises (Single arm)		2	8–10	
18 Posterior Back D.B. Raises (Single arm)		2	8–10	
37 Preacher Curls (Preacher bar or cables)	} Super Set	3	8–10	
20 Tricep Press-downs (V bar)			8–10	
24 Tricep Kick-backs	} One or the Other	2	8–10	
23 Tricep Dips (Dip Bar)		2	As many	
44 Standing Wrist Rolls		1 each way	40, 30, 25	
51 Gripper		2	As many	
52 Leg Extensions (Toes Pointed)	} Super Set	2	12–15	
54 Leg Curls			12–15	
53 Leg Extensions (Toes Back)	} Super Set	2	12–15	
54 Leg Curls			12–15	
60A Donkey Calf Raises (Straight)		2	20	
60B Donkey Calf Raises (In)		2	20	
60C Donkey Calf Raises (Out)		2	20	
61 Bench Sit-ups		2	As many	
62 Twisters		1	50 each way	

Stretch

Four-day Off-season Program
and
6-day Off-season Program

' Monday and Tuesday
then
Thursday and Friday

Example (Four-day):

Day One (Monday):   Chest, Shoulders, Triceps
Day Two (Tuesday):   Back, Biceps, Forearms, Legs (easier day)
Day Three (Thursday): Chest, Shoulders, Triceps (easier day)
Day Four (Friday):   Back, Bicep, Forearms, Legs

The Four-day Off-Season Program can easily be turned into a
Six-day Off-Season (as I do), by doing legs
on Wednesday and Saturday rather than Tuesday and Friday.

Example (Six-day)

Day One (Monday):   Chest, Shoulders, Triceps
Day Two (Tuesday):   Back, Biceps, Forearms (easier day)
Day Three (Wednesday): Legs (Day Two Legs Day) (easier day)
Day Four (Thursday):   Chest, Shoulders, Triceps
Day Five (Friday):   Back, Biceps, Forearms
Day Six (Saturday):   Legs (Day Four legs day)

Sunday Off

Third Program

Day One (Monday): Chest, Shoulders, Triceps

Stretch		Sets	Reps	Lbs.
1 Push-ups (Warm-up)		1		
3 Bench Press Supine		4	8–10	
6–8 Incline D.B. Press		3	8–10	
9 Cross-body Cable Pulls		3	8–10	
10 Military Press	Super Set	3	8–10	
12 Upright Rows			8–10	
16 Lateral Side D.B. Raises (Single Arm)	R-L, R-L, 30 Seconds	2	7	
17 Anterior D.B. Raises (Single Arm)	R-L, R-L, 30 Seconds		7	
18 Posterior Back D.B. Raises (Single Arm)	R-L, R-L, 30 Seconds		7	
27 Closed Grip Bench Press (Flat Supine)		4	8–10	
20 Tricep Press-downs (V Bar)	Super Set	4	8–10	
22 Tricep Bench Dips			As Many	
24 Tricep Kick-backs	One or the other	2	15	
25 Single-Arm Tricep Extensions		2	8–10	

Abs. 6" Leg Raises	15	6" Leg Raises	AB Crunches	¼ Sit-ups	30	Side Leg
25 Reps (M)	Sec.	20 Reps (M)	25 reps (S)	As many (F)	Sec.	Raises 10 Reps

	Sets	Reps
62 Twisters	1	50

Stretch before and after program

150

Day Two (Tuesday): Back, Biceps, Forearms, Legs (Easier day)

Stretch	Sets	Reps	Lbs.
28 Scapular Rolls	3	8–10	
29 Wide Grip Lat Pull-downs (Behind head)	4	10–12	
30 Wide Grip Lat Pull-downs (To chest)	3	10–12	
34 Bent Over Rows D.B.'s	3	10–12	
36 Hyperextensions (Lying down)	2	20	
35 Hyperextensions (Roman chair)	2	12–15	
43 Standing Preacher Curls	4	10–12	
41 Seated Incline D.B. Curls	3	10–12	
44 Standing Wrist Rolls	1 each way	40, 30, 25	
49 Wrist Abductions	2	As many	
50 Wrist Abductions	2	As many	
51 Gripper	2	As many	
52 Leg Extensions (toes pointed)	2	12–15	
53 Leg Extensions (toes back)	2	12–15	
54 Leg Curls	3	12–15	
57 Lunges	4	12–15	
59A Seated Calf Raises (Straight)	2	20	
59B Seated Calf Raises (In)	2	20	
59C Seated Calf Raises (Out)	2	20	
62 Twisters	1	50	

(36 and 35) } *One or the Other*

Stretch

Third Program

Day Three (Thursday): Chest, Shoulders, Triceps

		Sets	Reps	Lbs.
Stretch				
1 Push-ups (Warm-up)		1		
3 Bench Press Supine		4	8–10	
8 Incline D.B. Flys		3	8–10	
5 Decline Bench Press		3	8–10	
11 Seated Alternate D.B. Press		3	8–10	
16 Lateral Side D.B. Raises (Single Arm)	R-L, R-L, 30 Sec.	2	10	
17 Anterior D.B. Raises (Single Arm)	R-L, R-L, 30 Sec.	2	10	
18 Posterior Back D.B. Raises (Single Arm)	R-L, R-L, 30 Seconds	2	10	
19 Lying French Press		3	8–10	
21 Tricep Pull Downs (Rope)		2	8–10	
24 Tricep Kick-Backs	} One or the Other	2	15	
25 Single Arm Tricep Extensions		2	8–10	

Abs. 6″ Leg Raises	15	6″ Leg Raises	AB Crunches	¼ Sit-ups	30	Side Leg
25 Reps (M)	Sec.	20 Reps (M)	25 Reps (S)	As many (F)	Sec.	Raises — 10 Reps

		Sets	Reps	
62 Twisters		1	50	

Stretch

Day Four (Friday): Back, Biceps, Forearms, Legs

Stretch	Sets	Reps	Lbs.
28 Scapular Rolls Heavy Weight	2	20	
29 Wide Grip Lat Pull-downs (Behind head)	4	8–10	
30 Wide Grip Lat Pull-downs (To chest)	4	8–10	
31 Reverse Close Grip Pull-downs	4	8–10	
33 Single Handed Low Lat Pulls } *One or the Other*	3	6–8	
34 Bent Over Rows D.B.'s	2	6–8	
36 Hyperextensions (Lying down) } *One or the Other*	2	20	
35 Hyperextensions (Roman chair)	2	12–15	
37–38 Preacher Curls (Preacher Bench or Cables)	4	6–8	
39 Standing Alternate (Supinated) D.B. Curls	2	6–8	
40 Concentration Curls	2	6–8	
45 Wrist Curls } *Super Set*		8	
46 Reverse Wrist Curls		8	
47 Behind the Back Wrist Curls } *Super Set*	2	8	
48 Standing Reverse Wrist Curls		8	
49 Wrist Abductions } *Super Set*	2	8	
50 Wrist Abductions		8	
51 Gripper	2	50	
52 Leg Extensions (Toes Pointed)	2	12–15	
53 Leg Extensions (Toes Back)	3	12–15	
56 ¾ Leg Press	3	12–15	
60A Donkey Calf Raises (Straight)	2	20	
60B Donkey Calf Raises (In)	2	20	
60C Donkey Calf Raises (Out)	2	20	

Abs. 6″ Leg Raises	15	6″ Leg Raises	AB Crunches	¼ Sit-ups	30	Side Leg
25 Reps (M)	Sec.	20 Reps (M)	25 reps (S)	As many (F)	Sec.	Raises – 10 Reps

| 62 Twisters | 1 | 50 |

Stretch

Three-day Spring-training Program
(Only one option per body part)

No options on the middle or Wednesday
because this day is the easy day.

Example:

Monday (Day 1)   Wednesday (Day 2)   Friday (Day 3)

No option on this easy day

Do this program either after practice
or game or well before game time (early morning).

Stretch		Sets	Reps	Lbs.
3 Bench Press Supine	} Super Set	4	8–10	
32 Close Grip Lat Pull-Downs			8–10	
* 33 Single-handed Low-lat Pulls		2	8–10	
* 34 Bent Over Rows D.B.'s		2	8–10	
36 Hyperextensions (lying)	} Not both on the	2	20	
35 Hyperextensions (Roman chair)	same day	2	12–15	
13 Lateral D.B. Raises		2	10	
14 Anterior Front D.B. Raises (Double arm)		2	10	
15 Posterior Back D.B. Raises (Single arm)		2	10	
37 Preacher Curls (Cables)	} Not both on same day, pick one } Super Set	4	8–10	
Seated Preacher Curls (Pre-bench)			8–10	
20 Tricep Press-downs (V-bar)			8–10	
* 24 Tricep Kick-Backs		3	10–12	
* 25 Single Arm Tricep Pulleys		3	10–12	
44 Standing Wrist Rolls		1	40	
44 Standing Wrist Rolls		1	30	
44 Standing Wrist Rolls		1	25	
51 Gripper		2	As many (app. 40)	
52–53 Leg Extensions	Super Set } Two with toes pointed One with toes back	4	12–15	
54 Leg Curls			12–15	
59A Seated Calf Raises (Straight)		2	20	
59B Seated Calf Raises (In)		2	20	
59C Seated Calf Raises (Out)		2	20	

Abs. 6″ Leg Raises	15	6″ Leg Raises	15	AB. Crunches	20	¼ sit up	Side Leg
25 Reps (M)	Sec.	20 Reps (M)	Sec.	25 reps (S)	Sec.	as many (F)	raises (10 eachway)

62 Twisters	1	50

* Options

155

Fifth Program

Two-day-a-week In-season Program

A Maintenance Program

Monday and Thursday
or
Tuesday and Friday

Do the program after the game or early morning
before a night game.

Stretch	Sets	Reps	Lbs.
1 Push-ups (Warm-up)	3	8–10	
3 Bench Press Supine		8–10	
32 Close Grip Lat Pull-Downs } Super Set		8–10	
36 Hyperextensions (Lying)	2	20	
35 Hyperextensions (Roman chair) } One or the Other	2	12–15	
13 Lateral D.B. Raises	2	7	
14 Anterior Front D.B. Raises (Double arm) } Super Set		7	
15 Posterior Back D.B. Raises (Single arm)		7	
37 Preacher Curls (Cables) } One or the other	3	8–10	
Preacher Curls (Pre-bench) } Super Set		8–10	
20 Tricep Press-downs (V-bar)		8–10	
44 Standing Wrist Rolls	1	40	
44 Standing Wrist Rolls	1	30	
51 Gripper	1	As many (app. 40)	
52–53 Leg Extensions } Super Set { Two with toes pointed	3	12–15	
54 Leg Curls { One with toes back		12–15	
59A Seated Calf Raises (Straight)	1	20	
59B Seated Calf Raises (In)	1	20	
59C Seated Calf Raises (Out)	1	20	

Abs. 6″ Leg Raises	15	6″ Leg Raises	AB Crunches	¼ sit up	20	Side Leg Raises
25 Reps (M)	Sec.	20 Reps (M)	25 reps (S)	As many (F)	Sec.	As Many (M)

	Sets	Reps	
62 Twisters	1	50	

Stretch

Conclusion

Now that you have had an opportunity to look over what we consider to be one of the best workout plans ever developed for a baseball or potential baseball player, let's make a few general observations about the program: its use and its expectations.

There is, of course, no guarantee that this (or any other) program will make you into a major league baseball player. What the program is designed to do is maximize your potential. It will enable you to harness all of the physical capability for the game that your body has to offer.

If you do not have the desire or skill to become a professional player or the mental discipline to adhere to the program, you cannot expect to receive the maximum benefit.

However, if you follow the program regularly and perform its work correctly, you will be a fitter and healthier human being whether or not you ever play professional baseball at any level. That is a goal attainable for everyone.

Also, we wish to restate something we have said elsewhere: the program is not a bodybuilding program in the sense that it will give you an over-developed upper body, massive thighs, or other such things for impressing the guys at the gym or the girls at the beach.

It is what it says it is: a program to help you hone your body for the game of baseball, a game of particular muscle skills and endurance.

Further, bear in mind what has been said about the use of the program. A muscle has only 100 percent to give. Our purpose is to get that 100 percent from each muscle. But do not, ever, lift into pain or even into discomfort. We cannot stress this point too much or too often. Pain is a message. The message is simple: your muscles cannot handle the strain you are placing on them now. You must feel comfortable when you are lifting.

Do not be afraid to get professional help before you start the program or even if you do not fully understand some of the lifts. Don't guess. It is much better to ask than to run the risk of injury.

On a related subject, baseball (as mentioned above) is a game of endurance. You are expected to maintain your physical, mental, and emotional edge daily for 200 or more days each year. Although it is true that major league players get a day off every 19 days, they generally do some work in this program when they are off. At least, that is true of the Oakland Athletics for whom the program was designed.

There are other aspects to physical condition, too. Though this is not a book about diet or personal conduct, it should be obvious that these are important. There is a high degree of awareness today about the value of a healthy diet, and if you are or wish to be a professional athlete, it certainly makes good sense to look into this. Try to establish a diet that is healthy. Potato chips and hamburgers are fine once in a while, but the less often the better. Beware of foods with a lot of empty calories.

There are, of course, some baseball players (even in the major leagues) who smoke or drink alcohol (or both). Neither practice, however, is a good training habit. If you don't smoke or don't drink, don't start. If you do, try to quit. Failing that, limit your intake of tobacco or liquor as much as possible. Put yourself on a regimen. The self-discipline you develop will be of great help in dealing with the game of baseball. Many fine athletes have had trouble sustaining the level of concentration that baseball requires for the long season of the sport. Disciplining yourself with respect to these items will help you establish the proper frame of mind.

A word about steroids: don't use them.

Steroids may create the illusion of great gains in short periods of time, but they have a debilitating effect on your body chemistry, and in the long run you will be much worse off for having used them. The ultimate price you will have to pay is far, far greater than any short-term gain.

Also, baseball is not a game of large muscle. It is a game of strong, solid, durable muscle. Therefore, steroids have virtually no value even in the short term, if you are serious about baseball.

As to other drugs, nothing can be said here that hasn't already been said everywhere else. Only a fool becomes drug dependent. Fools have no chance to become stars in baseball or, probably, in any other aspect of life. Stay clean.

Having said all of that, we would like to wish you the best in using the program we have devised. It has worked very well for many major league players and we know, if followed precisely, it will work well for you.

While this program doesn't ensure you of a career in the major leagues, it will certainly enhance your chances of making it and ultimately succeeding in the game.